Author's biographical sketch

Columbia Hospital for Women, Washington DC, May 10, 1933 saw the birth of William A. Baxley. He grew up a "Government and Army brat, all around the USA." Then in early years worked in a West Virginia steel mill, was deck-hand on a Mississippi River towboat, map-drawing cartographer, oil-well roughneck in west Texas, and a New Hampshire State Mental Hospital extern, plus serving in the United States Marine Corps. ("Do stuff! Learn stuff!")

"As a young adult, I read Jack London, Ernest Hemingway, Joseph Conrad and other early twentieth-century realists; they convinced me that a major life-goal was to participate in the human drama as much as possible."

He graduated from Duke University twice, in 1955 with a BS in Civil Engineering (Phi Beta Kappa) and MD in 1962 (Alpha Omega Alpha Honor Medical Society) – now a fifth-generation medical doctor! Most of his professional career was spent on full-time clinical faculty at the University of Alabama Medical Center in Birmingham, retiring as Professor of Medicine-Cardiology in 1997.

Bax and wife Patricia Boswell run a small vacation-condominium/apartment rental business and live in Birmingham's South Side, the Metairie suburb of New Orleans, Northwest Florida's Emerald Gulf Coast at Seagrove Beach, and the Rocky Mountains in Big Sky, Montana. "Small places each, but all beautifully located."

Though author and co-author of over a hundred scientific publications, this is his initial incursion into popular writing: a self-portrait, with words instead of line and color, both fiction and non-.

3-29-20

To Charlie & Betsy Rackley with best wishes.

WCB

"Bax"

D1517724

LIFE – AND DEATH – IN THE HOSPITAL

A Memoir, Plus

By William A. Baxley, MD

Retired Professor of Medicine-Cardiology

School of Medicine, University of Alabama,

Birmingham, Alabama

NOTE TO LITERARY CRITICS, LIBRARIANS AND OTHERS CONCERNED WITH PUBLICATION CATEGORIES

This publication contains both non-fiction (memoir, Book I) and fiction (Book II), even poetry and screenplays (like some successful high-end American monthly magazines.) This combination may cause consternation to you. I suggest listing the title under both categories of *fiction* and *non-*, then with either asterisks (*) and an explanatory statement below, " * Contains also --," or simply this statement within the text.

With book publication currently undergoing vast change via electronic-books, now may be time to alter our rigid thinking re: format categories.

WAB

AUTHOR'S WARNING

You might not like this book.

It's different. And some of it is heavy.

Not everyone will like it.

But some will.

HISTORICAL NOTE

In 2010, the US Government passed the Affordable Medical Care Act ("Obamacare"). "For the better," say some; "For the worse," say others.

This book provides dramatic individual insights into medical care and medical education during that era before the law came into effect.

It's different now.

CONTENTS

* Screenplays written in style for readers, not for Hollywood.

PREFACE

Staff Cardiologist at the University of Alabama Medical Center for most of the years 1966 until retirement, 1997.

This could well be my future epitaph, but for me the years of "Life in the Hospital" actually began in 1960 with the clinical rotations of medical school, third and fourth years. Then from graduation in 1962 (Wow -- an MD!) until beginning junior-faculty at UAB in 1966, I was learning, post-graduate-style as Intern and Resident, then Cardiology Fellow (specialty trainee), all details about the heart and its problems.

[Funny story here: I skipped one of those years of "required" medical residency (was in a bit of a hurry). But then, years later as Instructor, teaching residents, in applying for Board Certification in Cardiology, "Why, Dr. Baxley! You're inadequately trained!" It took some explaining and convincing in addition to passing the required examination, but finally I won and they let me in. Even today I would advocate changes in specialty-training: my own area of coronary angioplasty would be better served with formal preparation in Radiology, Surgery and Anesthesiology instead of such Internal-Medicine subsets as Rheumatology, Oncology (cancer-treatment) and Hematology. But trying to modify established medical tradition is like trying to fight City Hall!]

During that entire epoch 1960-97, profound improvements evolved in the treatment of cardiac conditions. Catheterization with precise x-ray definition of structural defects and coronary artery blockages; intensive care units for heart attack victims; a whole variety of non-invasive (painless) imaging systems to peer inside of us; and an entire new world of medications, were some of the medical advances over those years. Add to that the astounding progress in cardiac surgery also!

For me the most thrilling new-comer was coronary angioplasty, or the "little balloon" (sometimes called, though not entirely correctly, the tiny roto-rooter) for non-surgical correction of coronary artery narrowings. For the first time it was possible to fix some of those dangerous and pain-causing obstructions without an open-chest operation. This development necessitated a whole different mind-set, plus a basic, emotionally-jarring identity change, to join the emerging subspecialty of Interventional Cardiology, especially for mid-career physicians like myself.

[For a well-written detailed history of interventional cardiology's development, read *Journey into the Heart* by David Monagan with David O. Williams, MD (Gotham Books, 2007). Particularly compelling was the meteoric rise of our procedure's charismatic inventor, Andreas Greunzig, MD. The book provides a chilling description of those final minutes at the controls of his private plane before a fatal crash in rural Georgia, stormy weather, the height of a spectacular career, age 46, October 27, 1985.

A tragic death, a true friend and hero of us coronary-angioplasty doctors worldwide.]

We performed the first coronary angioplasty in the State of Alabama at our University Hospital in 1982, and the technology raced ahead in the years to follow. Particularly important was development of the stent, a tiny spring "like that in your ball-point pen, only a bit larger," positioned inside the artery to prop it open while it heals. Our Interventional Unit was one of a world-wide group instrumental in improving stent technology. [Our Unit's director and my boss, Gary Roubin, MD PhD, while working at Emory University in 1987, after years of preliminary research, made history by placing a stent in an actual patient's coronary artery for the very first time. He has written an exciting history of this technology development: *The First Balloon Expandable Coronary Stent*, Amazon.com, 2015.]

Another important newcomer for us balloon-types was conducting Angioplasty Instruction Courses, utilizing the latest high-technology communication equipment internationally. We were one of a number of Medical centers staging these courses. Television cameras were set up in our procedure-rooms as well as in several others at such globally-diverse locations as Japan and Italy, to show details of a procedure in real-time. The audience of interventionalists relaxing in an auditorium would watch big-screens as live cases were performed, with split-screen imaging focused on the operating field and x-ray monitors. The spectators communicated questions and comments via microphone directly to moderators and the actual case operator. Procedures were performed sequentially at the various locations, one laboratory cleaning-up and preparing for next case, while live TV covered a procedure in another country. Obviously such courses required hard work in preparation and production, particularly for our head of Interventional Cardiology, Gary Roubin, MD PhD and second-in command Larry Dean, MD. The reality of these courses was compelling, as occasionally the angioplasty would fail on camera, the patient then taken abruptly to coronary bypass surgery (they always warned of this possibility before signing permits). Those four-day courses disseminated the newest techniques rapidly throughout the Angioplasty World.

Those were exciting years for all of us!

Retirement in 1997 required an abrupt emotional and physical transition into a more "normal" middle-class American lifestyle. This wasn't easy for me. However, as appreciating classical art in all forms has always been a major theme in my existance, I often recall lines of literature that suit a particular personal situation. So at this important life-juncture, I found a degree of solace in remembering those famous lines of English poet William Wordsworth (1770 – 1850):

"Though nothing can bring back the hour
Of splendor in the grass, glory in the flower,
We will grieve not, rather find
Strength in what remains behind."

So then I began a reflective retrospective odyssey over my past decades in the hospital. In addition to the profound technological evolution summarized above, it occurred to me that human drama, so intense and frequent at times on the medical scene, is mostly "lost in translation" and is rarely and inadequately transmitted into understandable forms for the lay population. Doctors in general are often not widely talented outside of our narrow focus onto medical science, further restricting any hospital-literary interface, and unfortunately some MDs don't relate too well with non-medical folk in general. This communication problem also goes in the other direction: I, like all doctors, have had experiences of explaining something medical to patient or family, speaking plainly, slowly, simply, repeatedly, only to then realize that they haven't understood – or maybe even totally misunderstood – my words. Sometimes during periods of stress, we humans hear only what we want to hear (or occasionally what we don't want to hear).

Medical-television dramas and a few movies attempt this task of revealing such dramatic intensity, but generally fall far short: unrealistic, silly, misleading are some adjectives that come at once to mind.

[Notable exceptions to this blanket criticism of acted medical-dramas are two movies: *MASH* (1970, written by Ring Lardner Jr., starring Donald Sutherland and Elliott Gould), and *The Hospital* (1971, written by Paddy Chayefsky, starring George C. Scott and Dianna Rigg). Though these films may seem unrealistic, they actually are not, particularly *Hospital*'s background milieu of daily life in a big city university-charity institution is dripping with reality.]

Many relevant non-fiction books selling today are agenda-driven, usually trying to convince the reader of terrible injustices in our American medical-care system. Then there are some scattered "pathographies" in print, wherein a physician ironically finds him-or-herself patient of the same type of disease he or she treats. The author-MD then proceeds to describe the emotional toll such affliction takes on patient and family. It doesn't take the proverbial Rocket Scientist, or in this case Rocket Psychologist, to see that such books or articles are often an attempt to assuage the author's guilt at not realizing earlier such emotional toll taken on his-or-her own patients. [See herein "The Physician as Patient" vignette for a different slant on this subject.]

Also there are some "heart-warming tales of courageous disease-fighting," or "Sensational! Astounding!" stories within the medical arena, some of which have a degree of merit.

This book avoids such standard categories, and hopefully the reader will find its candor and unaltered realism, utilizing a variety of literary platforms, to be engaging or even compelling, in both fiction and non - , and that it helps bridge today's medical-literary communication gap.

It all began as a doctor's memoir, but soon the autobiographical sketches progressed sequentially into medical fiction and thence to writings in various formats. The introductory tale, "The Doctor as Patient," and then all of "Autobiography" are totally true -- every word, every sentence, every paragraph, every chapter. Following that comes Fiction (the "plus" in my title), which by contrast is one-hundred percent imaginary, with credit clearly given for any borrowed character, writer or theme. A variety of literary formats is utilized for the different segments, each of which was carefully chosen to best express for the reader that particular dramatic episode of: Life and Death in the Hospital.

So symbolically I now hold out my hand with an invitation to you, the reader, to grasp it; I will then lead you on a journey through the world of The Hospital, with all of its colors from blinding light to total darkness – but be forewarned of varied emotional responses and new insights into the medical scene as gleaned throughout our journey.

This work has a carefully-orchestrated, almost musical, rhythm to its sequence. Thus "Dedication" and "Words --" set the tone, the milieu, the language of our trip; these two sections are as an entrance-hall to the main rooms of The Hospital.

After its opening tale, "Book One, Autobiography" recounts sequentially other true vignettes, revealing the stepping-stones of my path all the way from high school through faculty years and finally at age sixty-five, to retirement from the University of Alabama Medical Center and from all clinical, teaching and research activities.

Long ago I had trouble understanding and appreciating the abstract art of Spanish master Pablo Picasso. But then in Barcelona I viewed an extensive sequential display of his amazing works from childhood through early and then later adult years; so I began to understand: realism first (beautifully portrayed by him in landscapes and portraiture even as an adolescent), before later drifting into fantasy, all of the while maintaining the same feeling and intensity.

So after the realism-autobiography of Book One, we now step into the next room of that mansion, Hospital Life: Book Two, "Fiction" (another word for "Fantasy"). The four tales are grouped so, with increasing gravity, beginning with the humorous "Two-Eyed Girl" and finally culminating in the dark allegory "Intersection --." Then in "Terminus --" we return again to reality, though now in a lighter vein.

But wait, we're not through yet! The back-cover, "Rave Reviews!" is designed to send you off laughing, or at least smiling, as I release your hold and return to the book-front, "Hands," to greet our next reader.

DEDICATION

I am fortunate to have had many wonderful mentors throughout life, both as an ordinary citizen and academic medical doctor. This volume is respectfully dedicated to the four most important ones (now deceased):

-- **George Gale**, my high-school football coach (Shortridge, Indianapolis, IN, 1948-51), who taught me the basic rules of life.

The following three doctors were giants in their individual specialties, their names etched forever into the granite pillars of Medical Academe:

-- **Eugene A. Stead Jr, MD**, Professor and Chairman of Medicine at Duke University Hospital during my clinical-training years there, 1960-63.

-- **Harold T. Dodge, MD,** Professor of Medicine-Cardiology at University Hospitals in Seattle, Washington and then Birmingham, Alabama during my specialty training in cardiology and junior faculty years 1964-68. [See also "Engineering! Medicine!]

-- **John W. Kirklin, MD**, Cardiac Surgeon and Chairman of the Surgery Department, University of Alabama, Birmingham for most of my faculty years there from 1966. [See also "Words to Live by."]

Remembering also my great-great-grandfather, Henry Willis Baxley, MD (1803-76): clinician, educator, writer, world traveler, art critic and benefactor, who endowed the original Chair of Pathology at Johns Hopkins Medical School in Baltimore, MD.

Special thanks to long-time associate Theresa Sparks for manuscript advice and assistance; to college room-mate Edwin Michaels for the cover photo of my hands; to cousin-in-law Suzanne Pease for graphics and formatting; to wife Patricia Boswell for grammar review: and to scuba dive-buddies John Cooney, RN of the UK and Rodney Groomes, MD for refreshing my memory of those wild 1983 Red Sea adventures.

It was my distinct honor and privilege to serve in the United States Marine Corps. In return, one-fourth of profits from the sale of this book and all stage/screen productions therefrom are donated to the Marine Corps Scholarship Foundation (www.mcsf.org). This worthy organization assists Marines and their families in educational endeavors, particularly families of those Marines and Navy Medical Corpsmen serving with them who were killed in the line of duty.

Semper Fidelis!

FOR THE DOCTOR, WORDS TO LIVE BY

"Enter Herein, Only Ye Worthy Enough to Tend the Sick."
– Inscription over the entrance to an ancient Greek medical school

"I treated him. God cured him."
– Ambroise Paré (1510-90), French surgeon, on being praised by the King for "curing" a wounded soldier

"Life is short, the art [of medicine] long, judgment difficult and opportunity fleeting."
– Hippocrates, Ancient Greek physician

"The physician cures the patient's illness – rarely.
The physician alleviates the patient's symptoms – occasionally.
The physician comforts the patient – always."
– Fifteenth century European folk-saying

"Live your life in the medical wards."
– William Osler, MD (1849-1919), First Professor of Medicine at Johns Hopkins University, advising a medical student

"How to succeed in academic medicine? Listing the rules is easy; following them is hard.

- First, do pristine work. Seek perfection. There's no room for mistakes here.
- Second, work tirelessly, endlessly. Pay no attention to the clock or to the calendar. You didn't get into this business thinking it would be easy.
- Third, publish [in medical journals] everything [your research work], whether you like the results or not.

Follow these three simple rules and everything else will fall into place."

– John W. Kirklin, MD (1917-2004)
[See also "Dedication."]

"No greater opportunity, responsibility, or obligation can fall to the lot of a human being than to become a physician. In the care of the suffering, he needs technical skill, scientific knowledge, and human understanding. He who uses these with courage, with humility and with wisdom will provide a unique service for his fellow man and will build an enduring edifice of character within himself. The physician should ask of his destiny no more than this; he should be content with no less."

– Tinsley Harrison, MD (1900-78), who spent the major portion of his professional life as Professor and Chairman of the Department of Medicine, University of Alabama School of Medicine in Birmingham. [When these words were written, in contrast to today, almost all physicians were male.]

BOOK ONE

AUTOBIOGRAPHY

The Physician as Patient

By the 1970's, coronary by-pass surgery had been relatively well-refined and was generally safe and successful for appropriate patients. Most of those selectively chosen with anginal chest pain or its equivalent, such as exertional arm or jaw tightness, and occasionally even painless "silent ischemia," had symptom-relief and increased life expectancy. Because of the disease prevalence and popularity of this new procedure, operating rooms at times were almost overwhelmed and waiting lists extensive. When coronary-artery narrowings were severe but the patient asymptomatic at mild activity, a worrisome clinical situation had to be addressed: often such patients would be hospitalized for up to a week or so pre-operatively, being treated with a continuous strong intravenous blood thinner to keep the vessels open and so prevent an intervening catastrophic heart attack. These individuals would ambulate about the Coronary Care Unit in hospital garb, wearing their portable heart monitors and towing wheeled IV poles, trying to avoid boredom while awaiting their surgical dates.

We medical doctors, as all our fellow humans, may suffer from coronary artery disease or any of other numerous afflictions that can descend onto you or me.

So on a particular day in the late 1970s, we admitted an MD to our Coronary Care Unit, stable but with worrisome coronary blockages, to await his turn for surgery. Like the occasional others in a similar fix, he padded about the Unit, tethered to his monitor and pole. With a quiet, soft-spoken manner and quick, friendly smile, he soon established himself to other patients, families and staff as a regular member of the Unit. Though a physician, he was never obtrusive, but instead consoling, understanding and comforting. He had a way of reflecting compassion and an awareness of the emotional toll being taken on the patients and families about him, never expressing a scientific opinion or questioning a clinical decision. As Unit Rounds took place each morning with doctors and nurses sequentially reviewing each patient's status and plan, he stood silently to the side of the group. With rounds completed, he would visit every patient and family at the bedside, not scientifically medical but as a fellow human, suffering too with a similar affliction. He chatted informally with Unit Staff – nurses, technicians, students, secretaries, doctors, assistants – but only during moments of their brief respite from chores. He slept little, and this human-to-human communication took place at all hours, day and night, each work-shift.

None of the staff, patients or families realized over the passage of days, his growing importance and closeness to them. The fact that he was both doctor and patient seemed to deepen this bonding.

Finally, a week after his hospital admission, time arrived for his own coronary by-pass operation.

After surgical attendants helped him onto the gurney for transport to the preparation room, he paused, "Wait, just a moment – do you mind? Please ask any of the Unit Staff available to come for a minute. "

All of those not urgently occupied assembled.

His eyes were moist, but he still had his wide smile and unhalting voice as he addressed them: "I just wanted to tell you all – I've been a close part of your group for a week now – just to tell you how good you are scientifically, and I'd have to say, compassionate. You are thoughtful and considerate in every way, working with these severely ill patients and their close ones. Now I know I'm not going to make it, so I just wanted to thank you all and say goodbye."

The response to his address was universal:

"Don't talk like that! You're in great shape."

"Stop it! No pessimism please. We'll visit you post-op."

"That's silly for you to say, Doctor."

But in the following hours, an air of anxiety and unrest pervaded throughout the Unit: furtive glances, worried looks, frequent time checks, no soothing background music now.

"He should be out soon -- "

"I hope he's okay -- "

When a surgeon or any physician contemplates a patient-procedure having an element of danger, he or she carefully determines the expected risk. Age, general health condition and specific organ status such as that of lungs and kidneys, are evaluated. For heart surgery, the strength of the cardiac muscle and the number and location of blockages are important variables. The doctor considers all of these factors, uses the best judgment possible in prediction, and then describes to the patient the chances of a successful operation and recovery. In modern times these odds often well exceed ninety-five percent, and the patient usually says, "Okay! Safe. Go ahead."

But for that remaining small percent, there is no survival.

When notice of his intra-operative death flashed back to the Unit, the result was electric, palpable, devastating.

"No! No!"

"I can't believe it!"

"Not that nice doctor!"

4

All Unit Staff not involved in immediate patient care raced into the nurses work room. Tears flowed freely, though there was no loud outcry. Phone calls to the evening and night shift personnel quickly followed. One nurse recalled sadly, "He even predicted his own fate before leaving here -- must have had a premonition." Another, a male, weeping bitterly, explained simply, "I can't take this anymore. I'm turning in my notice." But the remaining staff cried; grieved; consoled one another; then dried their eyes, took deep breaths and went back to their duties of caring for the severely ill, knowing that this would not be the last deeply-felt death to cross the portals of their Coronary Care Unit.

> "No man is an island,
> No man can live alone.
> So ask not for whom the death-bell tolls –
> It tolls for thee."
> – John Donne
> (English Poet, 1572-1631)
> (Paraphrased)

THE EARLY YEARS

"White Crosses on Their Football Helmets! Wow!"

A rather unheralded start, with even some adolescent-comedy sprinkled in, but nevertheless, in looking back, a first step on that long, long path.

It was during the autumn of my senior high-school year. I was lounging on our sofa reading the newspaper -- a sleepy Sunday afternoon. Sitting nearby in his favorite easy chair was my father, a good dad, both parents steering me through the fog and around the potholes of teen age.

"Son, a good education is important these days. You should go to college next year. Do you know where you might want to go?"

Well, I knew I liked to play football and chase after girls, and I was pretty good at mathematics; at the time, that was just about the extent of my thinking about life, the future, and worldly topics in general.

"Gee, don't know – hadn't really thought about it."

"Why don't you give it some consideration and let me know. Then we'll discuss it and see what we can work out for you to go to college."

"Okay."

So I resumed reading the sports page.

And there was a large, action, color-photograph from a Duke University football game – and the Duke players wore dark blue helmets with two white stripes, one lengthwise from forehead to neck, the other ear to ear, forming a white cross on top. Totally different from all other teams! Sooo cool! Utterly awesome! White crosses on blue backgrounds, just like the crusaders and knights of old!

Then I said the word *Duke* to myself. Spectacular! Short and crisp!

Unlike In-di-an-a Un-iv-er-sit-y, or Sou-thern Meth-o-dist, two other colleges mentioned in the paper.

So there and then I announced, "Dad, I want to go to Duke!"

I spent nine years at Duke University in Durham, North Carolina: four in college, four in medical school and one in medical internship.

I married a Duke girl (first marriage).

My oldest son graduated from Duke.

All because their football players had white crosses on their helmets!

A Glass of Scotch Leads to a Career
Spanning Thirty-five Years

The second step on that long road was a bit more focused, still with some humor.

 So there I was, a senior engineering student at Duke University, a member of the United States Marine Corps Reserve, to serve two years active duty after graduation (this during the peaceful interval between our Korean and Vietnamese wars). College studies were interesting, though I was unsure of an ultimate career direction, in fact not thinking about it much. I made excellent grades and enjoyed classes -- a happy life-interval: brain food (actually enjoyed assignments!), pretty girls, the Sigma Chi Fraternity, afternoon physical work-outs.

My parents had recently relocated to Huntington, West Virginia, where Dad was manager of a large hospital, our house nearby. Next door lived a young general surgeon, a friendly outgoing fellow. With few buddies there, I soon hooked up with him socially. Whenever home during holidays, we two would visit a local bar for beer and conversation. He was forever interested in what we college students were up to -- politically, socially, sports-wise, music-wise, and other-wise. Occasionally he would suggest that I "come up to the hospital and watch an operation. You might find surgery intriguing." In response, I would *think*, but in typical adolescent fashion, not *say*, "Oh, gross! All that blood and guts. I'd probably faint!" Instead I would simply demur, "No thanks."

But, one night at the bar, as chance -- or *fate* -- would have it, there was no more beer!

"Have you ever tried Scotch?" my friend asked.

"No."

"Perhaps now is the time to try it."

9

"Well, er, okay, I guess so – "

Later he invited, "Come up to the hospital in the morning. I'm doing a gallbladder. You can scrub in and see what it's all about."

So under the influence of my initial experience with hard alcohol, I agreed – hesitantly.

Next early AM I arrived in surgery, followed instructions, donned the appropriate sterilized apparel including mask and cap, scrubbed hands and arms, then into gown and gloves. They directed me to a position beside the surgeon as "assistant." (!!) Others on the team were the scrub-nurse across the operating table from us, primarily for handling instruments; a circulator for non-sterile duties; and the anesthetist seated at our patient's head.
I was slightly less than terrified.

When all was ready, abdomen scrubbed and draped, the patient nicely asleep, the surgeon took his scalpel and made an initial incision through the skin, parallel to and just below the right rib cage, about five inches long. Then using instruments called "clamps," which looked like small thin long-nosed pliers, but used in reverse, to open tissue rather than clasping something, he deepened the incision through superficial fat and the four layers of abdominal muscle. This created a progressive opening, parallel to the muscle fibers of each layer, " -- rather than cutting across them. This is less traumatic and hastens healing." He avoided large blood vessels, tying off any small bleeders with thin silk sutures while controlling capillary oozing with gentle pressure of sponges (small cotton pads). Then the scalpel again to incise the fibrous peritoneum lining of the abdominal cavity, exposing the liver's edge. Below it nestled the gallbladder, a thumb-sized digestive organ not truly essential and here infected. Cautiously tying off its stem, he then cut it free and carefully lifted it away with instruments, placed it in a pan for pathological examination and handed the pan to – me! Now backing out, he placed sutures in each anatomical layer he had opened, approximating tissue edges first and then tying the sutures, "just firm enough to hold the layers in place but not so tight as to obstruct capillary blood flow, which would impede healing and even might invite infection." Finally came skin sutures to remain ten days, a sterile dressing and then lastly discontinuing anesthesia.

In terms of my daunted "blood and guts", blood loss onto the sponges was less than several ounces, and the only "guts" visible was the pink-grey shiny surface of the colon, seen as it coursed transversely under the liver's edge.

For the first time in my life, I was absolutely, totally shocked! I was astounded! Immediately, instantly, I knew what I was going to do the rest of my life. This was life! This was *reality*, not the games and silliness that seem to dance about us endlessly in our daily existence. Science and compassion rolled into one. The true human drama! My life's destiny without question.

Later I sat on the curb behind our house and stared blankly, chin in hands. "It is now not a questions of what to do with the future, but how to do it, how to get into medical school." That would require a return to college part-time for a year of biology, advanced chemistry and other prerequisite courses, after two years of active duty in the United States Marine Corps.

I began Medical School at Duke University in the fall of 1958.

I have never regretted my decision.

A Doctor's Footprints

Medical school application generally requires at least three years of college, including specific required "pre-med" courses. Admission committees of faculty members are intensely selective, studying past accomplishments of each applicant and then interviewing most, attempting to choose the best qualified from a variety of perspectives, not only scholastic. (In my case, I read where on average, only one in ten applicants was accepted, so I applied to ten different schools!) So once enrolled, most students then graduate; this is the American style of medical education. In contrast, many other countries, including European, are less selective in admissions, with larger first-year classes which are then pared down sequentially by difficult examinations along the way.

Following four years of study comes graduation; he or she (now an MD!) then progresses through a number of hospital and clinic, post-graduate, on-the-job training years termed PG-1, PG-2, etc. as intern, resident, and fellow. Depending upon specialty pursuits, this can reach as many as eight years after graduation. Each annual advance entails additional clinical responsibility on the chosen team, plus a few more dollars on the fairly meager pay check. Particularly in university hospitals, fellows, the most specialized of trainees, also regularly participate in clinical research; projects involving patients as opposed to basic research strictly in the laboratory.

So each year presents the student or young doctor* with its own unique interface onto the stage of hospital drama, as we shall see in the following dialog.

*Though after so many years of training, the doctor may not be exactly "young" anymore!

In the Beginning –

Before our modern "high-tech" era, the first year of medical school was devoted to learning human *normality* in detail: anatomy (both gross, meaning to the unaided eye, and microscopic), physiology (what each organ-system does), biochemistry, psychology and multiple related sub-topics. On day-one, the student is introduced to a stark, grim reminder of human mortality: the cadaver. Over the course of many months, these formaldehyde-embalmed bodies are tediously dissected by students according to carefully prescribed protocols. In recent years, ingenious computerized study-aids augment the anatomy course, and sadly some schools now consider abolishing cadaver use altogether. But this actual human body adds an immediate and profound sense of reality and intensity to the student – no light-hearted banter now!

Our 1958 first-year class predated the computer age. But that didn't stop Duke's Professor of Anatomy, Joseph Markee, PhD, from being way ahead of his time with teaching-aids. Earlier, he with assistants alone in their anatomy laboratory, had set up a movie-camera complete with lights and "technicolor" film, focused on sequential body-sections of a cadaver. He would make a prescribed scalpel-incision, dissect free the individual underlying anatomic structures, and then color-code them with paint, their natural formaldehyde-treated hue a sickly orange-mauve-grey. Nerves were painted yellow, veins blue, arteries red. He then folded the structures and skin back into their natural or untouched positions. Now to start the camera, both video and audio, rolling. He next assumed a position beside the cadaver and, delivering his lecture, acting as if he were making the initial incision and then dissection, revealing on film the underlying body-parts clearly, in all their obvious color-coded glory.

So each Saturday morning we began class with his movie-presentation depicting what we would perform the next week on our assigned cadavers in the main anatomy laboratory, generally four students per body, with instructors circulating. [Dr. Markee was a medical scientist, not a poet – pretty factual. However there seem exceptions to everything. He had written our Human Anatomy Laboratory Workbook which we used daily, and who among us students could ever forget that colorful, almost romantic, opening line to his chapter, "The Female Pelvis": "The female pelvis may be likened unto a box." Shakespeare meets Gynecology 101!]

This format mixed with other integrated lecture and laboratory courses, geared toward human normality, provided an exciting first year, even absent contact with patients.

Thus having spent the first medical school year focusing on the normal human body, it was now time to study *abnormality* in detail – those illnesses and injuries that send us to the doctor: so enter the second year.

The term pathology means the study or science of disease and injury – the departure from human normality, particularly in terms of bodily structure. A related term, pathophysiology, is the science of the subsequently altered organ function.

The word *autopsy* may conjure up gruesome thoughts to non-medical folk, yet in many respects it is simply a surgical operation performed after death. Its primary purpose is defining conclusively and in detail the exact cause of demise. Organs and tissue samples are examined grossly and microscopically; blood tests are performed and various materials may be cultured for evidence of bacterial or viral infection. Finally, the bodily remains are disposed of according to family wishes.

Yet in addition to determining death-cause, a second purpose is often most important: that of a teaching exercise. Any student or young doctor assisting at a post-mortem examination or later studying the results learns significant lessons in medical science therefrom: correlating the medical history and other clinical data with autopsy findings. These lessons are particularly impressive if the body is that of his-or-her previous patient, though this combination of events may prove emotionally disturbing to some, especially if early in their medical careers.

Unfortunately, in recent years as medical malpractice lawsuits have burgeoned, autopsy-permission requests to families of deceased patients have dwindled. Fears of finding some undiagnosed "cause", which then might trigger a malpractice-suit with all of its devastating consequences, have greatly blunted this important educational procedure. Previously these examinations were routinely sought and family-permission often granted (at no expense to them).

At the start of our second school year 1959-60, every hall in Duke Hospital's Pathology Department was lined floor-to-ceiling with wide shelves filled with large, covered, numbered pots. This collection contained the preserved, relevant anatomic specimens from every autopsy performed at the institution since its inception in 1925. Close at hand were file cabinets containing the corresponding reference numbers, microscopic tissue slides and clinical data including case histories, physical examination findings and laboratory data, but no identifying names or dates. An old black-and-white photograph of our then-young-appearing Professor of Pathology, Wiley Forbus, MD, hung nearby. In it he wore rubber gloves and black apron, an assistant near, both behind the autopsy table with corpse; an inscription below recorded a decades-earlier date, and, "The first autopsy at this institution revealed that the patient died of acute hemorrhagic pancreatitis."

At 1 PM each weekday our second-year class of sixty assembled into a small, steep, arena-shaped conference room adjacent to the autopsy laboratory for "Pathology Round Up." Professor Forbus sat silently, immobile and stern-looking, in center-stage, facing four empty chairs; a hushed, anxious air prevailed. He would then read the names of

15

four randomly-chosen students from his list. As the four climbed down and sat facing him, an audible sigh of relief emanated from those remaining. The four selected would then be grilled orally by the professor for the next hour concerning the previously-assigned subject, the grilling occasionally interrupted by questions or invited comments from the stands.

Following this traumatic hour, the four chosen breathed their relief-sighs and wiped sweaty foreheads.

The class then divided into small groups with instructors and proceeded into work-rooms containing pots, slides and clinical data, chosen as examples of the disease or injury currently under study.

There we remained for the next three hours.

Each group first reviewed the clinical history, physical signs and ancillary data of a previous, actual, suffering individual person. Then we held in our gloved hands for examination the diseased or injured organ and visualized the projected microscope tissue slides. Examples included such cases as a golf-ball sized stomach cancer blocking outflow, with our noting that this patient had presented to the doctor with severe vomiting and weight loss, or examining a spleen (cucumber-shaped blood-organ tucked up under the left rib-cage), fatally ruptured by a kick to the abdomen during some bar-room brawl. This sequence produced an intimate association of true patient-symptom-disease, deeply affecting each of us medical students.

Such an instruction routine, plus our assisting at all autopsies on a rotating basis, was followed for the entire second school-year; today it would be considered old-fashioned, those pots being supplanted by high-technology, color-coded, three-dimensional teaching aids. But for us it worked, in large part because of a simple reality: true hands-on, human tissue examinations by students.

Indeed, ours was the last class to benefit thus; at the end of a long outstanding academic career, Dr. Forbus then retired. That spring as the school-year was concluding, following Duke Hospital's final-ever "Pathology Round-Up," our class delivered a prolonged standing ovation, even moist eyes, for that wonderful strict-but-fair professor, bringing forth the only occasion I ever saw him smile.

So Pathology, with its close-sister Pathophysiology, dominated our second-year study. Also there were morning courses including physical examination as practiced on each other, studies in x-ray and other imaging techniques, and the laboratory abnormalities resulting from illness or injury.

But still no living-patient contact! At year's end we were as race horses, breathlessly waiting for the gate to open: anticipation for the next – *clinical* – year.

(We had been introduced to death tangentially in terms of cadavers and autopsies, but had not yet encountered the death of a patient.)

Death (Part One)

"I, Antonius Block, a Knight returning home from the Crusades, am playing chess with Death."

-- The Seventh Seal, 1957 film by Ingmar Bergman

Finally!!

Thus, traditionally at that time, only third and fourth medical-school years were clinical, interacting with actual patients as part of a ward or out-patient team -- the lowest-ranked member, often referred to as a "gopher", as in, "Hey you! Student! Go for the x-rays." The object was to continue, now in a practical manner, the basic lessons of the first two years.

So on day-one of my third medical-school year I was ready and anxious to begin. Checked myself in the mirror: short white student's jacket with stethoscope, pen, notebook and "little black bag" of small tools used in physical examination. Then at the appropriate time I dutifully marched up to my assigned medical ward. Entering the Doctors' (!) Work Room, I introduced myself to the resident, who was busy writing in patients' charts. Rather brusquely he instructed, "Go listen to Ms __'s heart, Room __. She has an interesting murmur." (heart sound sometimes indicating disease). I proceeded to her room, knocked; no answer. I cautiously entered. A middle-aged female lay in bed, head rolled up, breathing quietly, eyes closed. Introducing myself, then, "I'm here to examine your heart with my stethoscope." No answer. So I listened intently over the first prescribed cardiac area of the left anterior chest, as we students had practiced on ourselves: "lub-dub, lub-dub, lub-dub," (the normal heart sounds, usually repeated regularly every second or so.) But then a pause – then, "lub-dub, lub-dub." I strained to hear a murmur, as we had learned on audio recordings, but couldn't hear any. Then the sounds seemed to grow softer. I moved to the next prescribed area of the chest, the sounds still softer and seemed to slow somewhat. I moved to the third location; still the same. I removed the 'scope from my ears, checked it and progressed on to the fourth and final chest-location and listened intently – the lub-dub was now quite soft. I removed my stethoscope, checked it again, re-applied it, concentrating hard. A few very soft sounds, then silence. Disappointed and feeling totally dumb and inadequate, I slouched slowly back to the

Doctors' Workroom and Resident. "Something wrong with either my ears or the 'scope. Not only do I hear no murmur, I hear no heart sounds at all." He arose, and after a few unkind words blasting "inept medical students," accompanied me to her room.

The woman was dead.

Unknowingly I had heard her final heart beats! She had died precisely while I was examining her. My first actual patient! After two years of study and anticipation – this!!

Such was my introduction to clinical medicine.
This dark specter, *death*, had been standing there beside me, laughing at my student-ignorance and I hadn't recognized her.

She was to follow me for the next thirty-seven years, as she does all physicians who attend severely ill patients – often lurking in the wings, remaining silent for weeks, other times a quick and unannounced appearance, occasionally proclaiming her presence and plan well in advance; even she, herself, on rare occasions, weeping, as she delivers her strike.

"Life and death in the Hospital"

Surgery

The third and fourth medical school years involve a series of hospital or out-patient clinic six-week rotations in various specialties – Internal medicine, obstetrics, surgery, pediatrics, etc., and sometimes electives in subspecialties such as orthopedic surgery or hematology.

It was during my senior year, general surgery rotation. An operation was planned relatively urgently on a middle-aged male with an expanding abdominal aortic aneurysm (swelling of the main blood vessel, with high probability of fatal rupture if uncorrected). Such aortic repair was risky and complex because of the large number of arteries arising from it, supplying multiple vital organs. (In years following, better preventives and safer treatment options evolved.)

I was to second-assist. In final preparation I sat on the bed beside the patient, reviewing once more our treatment plan, no one else present. To my surprise, he reached over and started stroking my thigh in a most inappropriate manner, a definite homosexual move. I drew away from him and soon discreetly concluded the visit.

The operation was long and difficult. Our anesthesiologist, charged with two duties, kept the patient painlessly asleep, but also utilized a variety of fluids and medications to maintain optimal total-body physiologic function while the surgeon did his repair work. She periodically recited various parameters of vital importance – arterial oxygenation, cardiac-circulatory status and multiple others.

Clearly these parameters reflected a slow general physiologic deterioration.

Then, "I'm having trouble keeping up with him, Sir."

Finally after an extended pause, "I'm sorry, Sir. We're losing him. I'm maxed out. I'm sorry, Sir," and she recited parameters confirming her assessment.

The attending surgeon stopped his work, sighed, stared deeply into the eyes of each team member, removed his gloves and mask. Departing the operating room, he instructed the anesthesiologist, "Discontinue support," and to me, "Close up."

I used good surgical technique in closing; first the blood vessels, then the fibrous peritoneum lining the abdomen, several muscle layers, superficial adipose and finally skin. As I did so, I thought, "Well, my friend, awhile back you made inappropriate advances on me, and now I'm sewing up your lifeless body. Is this irony, sarcasm, fate, or justice?"

Humor??

In dealing with patient deaths, one of the most unpleasant tasks for any doctor is notifying family or friends, particularly if the event is sudden or unexpected or of a young person. We encounter the entire spectrum of human emotion in response: grief, rage, collapse, denial, prayer, to name a few, but -- humor?

A legend concerning the Emergency Department at Duke University Hospital circulated during the 1960's while I was in clinical training there. I have heard it repeated from so many different sources over such an extended period of time that I suspect truth:

A severely injured woman was brought in urgently by her husband. Immediate and proper treatment was to no avail; the woman died soon after admission, there in the trauma-treatment room. It was the intern, a new MD, who, even though shaken by the event, was given the sad task of notifying the husband.

He did this as gently and succinctly as possible.

Then the husband looked up and, "Don't take it so hard, Doc – I've got her insured!"*

* I love telling this story to friends in the insurance business!

Oops!!

"Cheynne-Stokes respiration" [Medical phenomena are often named for those individuals who first described them.] is a particular type of breathing pattern during sleep, often requiring prolonged observation to recognize. Our normal respirations are usually regular, fast or slow depending on activity and other factors (unless interrupted by a cough or sneeze). But with Cheynne-Stokes, breathing together with heart-rate and blood pressure, rhythmically slows – markedly, even stopping transiently – and then over the next few minutes speeds up dramatically.

This repeated phasic pattern is usually termed abnormal, as a type of breathing disorder, but it can occasionally be observed in asymptomatic older folk or simply those mildly sedated.

While I was first-year medical resident, we admitted an elderly male with advanced, through barely symptomatic, cancer. (In those years past, doctors tended to hospitalize patients for diagnostic evaluation, rather than the cheaper but less convenient practice of out-patient clinic use, as done today.) His second night on the ward happened to be one of my few nights off, a colleague-resident covering my duties. Toward midnight the nurse called my cover, stating that our cancer patient had died in his sleep. She requested he come certify the death, then notify family. He arrived, examined the patient, concurred, and sat down in the work station to write a death note in the chart before calling family. Then the nurse came rushing in, quite excited, "Doctor, come quick!" He raced back to the elderly man, who was sleeping, not dead! This was not religious "resurrection"; this was Cheynne-Stokes. Both doctor and nurse had been fooled by a brief interval of no pulse, no breathing.

On rounds next AM, I noticed in the patient's chart the beginning of a note which had then been crossed through. I called and questioned my last-night's cover; he sheepishly explained the events.

Then I asked the patient how he had slept the previous night.

"I seemed to have slept exceptionally deeply last night, thank you, Doctor."

Later he was discharged home and spent several months with family before – actually – dying.

Sometimes Nature plays jokes on us all!

Medical Student
Clinical Rotations

"Anesthesiology? -- Well, Probably Not –"

During my senior medical-school year, like most fellow students, I considered various specialties for future training. Anesthesiology was one of several that appealed to me – precise and scientific, yet at times dramatic; features I liked. So I took a six-week anesthesiology elective, working mostly in surgical settings as the lowest-ranking member in their patient-care and educational activities. I was a good student, worked and studied hard and even enjoyed the long hours in pre-operative, intra-operative and "post-op" patient care. In-between cases I attended conferences, and in-between the in-betweens was library-time for texts and journals. But, I had major flaws: was arrogant, overconfident, cocky, and basically full of myself; only later did the realities of life in the hospital cause the word *humble* to creep into my vocabulary.

Toward the end of the elective I convinced my attending anesthesiologist for permission to administer the anesthesia for a surgical procedure, "with staff supervision, of course."

Of course.

It was minor hand-repair surgery, not a difficult or protracted operation, though it did require brief general anesthesia, the patient asleep. I sat at the patient's head, carefully attending to the intra-venous fluids and to the oxygen-mixture mask over his mouth and nose; this type of procedure did not require intubation of the windpipe. I had calculated all parameters and doses carefully; three anesthetics were utilized, one inhalation through the mask and two intra-venous.

My attending stepped out of the operating room momentarily, but no need to worry – I was on top of everything!

The two surgeons sat on little stools beside the patient's arm, which was outstretched, supported and draped, palm up and scrubbed.

"Anesthesiology ready to begin the operation?" one of them asked me.
Now my correct response should have been, "One moment, Sir, until my

attending returns and checks everything out." Instead, arrogance and over-confidence won out: "YES, SIR!"

The chief surgeon took the scalpel and made the initial superficial skin incision across the patient's palm, from base of thumb to little finger. The patient immediately sat bolt upright on the operating table, scattering instruments and sterile drapes in all directions! He was anesthetized just enough so that he didn't utter a sound or open his eyes, but there was suf-ficiently generalized discomfort felt to cause bodily withdrawal. The looks those two surgeons gave me graphically defined the word *glare*. I quickly opened all three anesthetic agent flow-rates full, and the patient instantly swooned back onto the table ("just like in a comic movie," I would later recall.)

About that time our attending anesthesiologist returned. "Everything okay?"

"Well Sir, we got off to a little ragged start, but now we're fine."

Then in the recovery room post-operatively, my reactive and zealous use of anesthetics caused a slight delay in the patient's awakening; during this interval I had to rhythmically squeeze the airflow-bag to his oxygen mask, to insure adequate ventilation until he fully awakened and was normally breathing on his own.

After I finally arrived home from the hospital late that night, fore-arms sore from the protracted bag-squeezing, I looked into a mirror and spoke aloud, "Well, Baxley, maybe you should consider some other specialty besides anesthesiology!"

[As a post-segment comment, in my thirty-five years of medical academe I have never once observed a patient harmed by the actions of any stu-dent or doctor-in-training; however, I have observed patients harmed by improper actions of staff physicians (including myself), nurses, nurse-anesthetists and various other medical assistants and technologists, some of which later progressed to the courtroom.]

Engineering! Medicine!

Stroll about any large university medical complex these days
and you will discover a Department of Bioengineering. Further
investigation therein reveals research, development and educational
projects involving such areas as heart pacemakers; artificial limbs and
joints; monitors of heart rhythm and other physiologic parameters;
improvements in CAT-scans and various new imaging systems to
investigate our insides with a minimum of risk and inconvenience; and
even circulatory-assist devices including mechanical hearts.

It wasn't always so.

Reviewing the history of science shows that most important
discoveries through the ages resulted from curiosity and an inquisitive
bent by exceptionally smart individuals willing to discard previous
perceptions. Of course chance, together with the ethical, social and
even religious milieu have played important roles – note the eras of
scientific advancement during both the Renaissance and the Age of
Enlightenment (1700's). In contrast to simple scientific curiosity,
occasionally practical problem-driven quests have resulted in
monumental discoveries: Thus in ancient times, the King of Syracuse,
Sicily, wished to learn if his crown was pure gold or had been illegally
diluted with cheaper metals. He sought the famed scientist Archimedes
(287-212 BC), who reflecting over the problem while reclining in his
bathtub, envisioned and later quantitated the buoyancy principle which
permanently bears his name: any object in a fluid is buoyed up with
a force equal to the weight of the fluid displaced by said object. This
simple formula, in addition to ultimately answering the king's question,
is the mathematical basis for every ship, including submarines, designed
by marine engineers since that time.

But the most far-reaching discoveries for engineering in my opinion
were made by the Englishman Sir Isaac Newton (1643-1727). He
gave us differential and integral calculus (instantaneous quantitation

of varying space-time and other complex relationships); the exact definition of gravity; and most importantly this simple truth; for moving objects, force equals mass multiplied by acceleration ($F = MA$). This little formula has allowed us to reach Mars, as well as permitting design of everything man-made that moves. (We won't even get into computers and the invention of microchips, or to atomic energy, the legacy of Albert Einstein.)

For us in the medical specialty of cardiology, the stand-out discovery was made by the English physician William Harvey (1578-1657). For eons before his 1628 scientific paper "Exercditatio Anatomica de Circulations Sanguinis," doctors had various incorrect notions about human circulation; a popular one was that the heart pumped blood in a back-and-forth or oscillating manner. (In some lower biological species, this type of circulatory-mechanism indeed exists.) But Harvey made an exceedingly simple observation that defied tradition, which anyone with access to another person having large visible arm veins can easily repeat: he simply pressed one finger over such a vein, and then with another finger "milked" the blood from it up toward the body. He thus was looking at a collapsed segment of vein with a finger pressing at each end of the segment, keeping it empty. He noted that if he released the distal finger only, the vein-segment quickly dilated and filled with blood, but if instead he released the proximal (closer to the body) finger only, the vein-segment remained collapsed. This demonstrated clearly that blood in veins flows only in one direction – back to the heart. Centuries of false theories trounced at once! This little observation lead to the entire truth; blood leaves the left-heart via arteries, then circulates everywhere through capillaries and thence to veins where it returns to the right-heart and then through the lungs back to the left side of the heart.

So one appealing concept of practical scientific philosophy is this: there are three basic spheres of scientific endeavors, one more pure and two more practical as applied to the human situation. The first, true science, is represented by geniuses such as Isaac Newton and Albert

Einstein, who quantitate the basic tenets of nature. The other two spheres, engineering and medicine, utilize these basics for the benefit of mankind: engineers to reshape the world around us, and medical doctors to utilize science for our own bodily health (medical science less exact than engineering, the human body containing an endless number of mathematical variables, and the ethics of experimentation another constraint).

Only recently has bioengineering emerged as the overlap of these two practical applications of pure science.

In 1962 I was a Duke Hospital intern, fresh out of medical school, on the first rung of the post-graduate education ladder. It was a tough life. On many of the six-week differing clinical rotations, there was never a day off and only two nights free weekly (Thursday and Saturday nights one week, Friday and Sunday nights the next, etc.) We lived in the hospital otherwise, this in contrast to today's Federal-law mandated much easier house-staff schedules. But such a grind provided spectacular platforms for medical learning: we were there, participating, whenever critical treatment-decisions had to be made, and then the patient's improvement, or worsening, followed. But this "almost-24/7/52" grind took a toll on students and house-staff. During my first three clinical years, one event each year still remain in my memory: one, a house officer during work simply stated, "I quit," gathered his belongings, walked out of the hospital and we never saw him again. Another year an intern suffered severe acute depression and had to be removed from duties, and then the third and most tragic, a suicide. One of these events happened as I was just completing a most-difficult six week rotation, and "Baxley, sorry, we've had to rework the schedule, you'll have to cancel your departure and continue on for another six weeks." Oh, no, a full three months with never a day off and only rare free nights!

And the Sabbath was no exception to this harsh routine. Our weekly "Sunday School" had no religious basis – rather a series of medical lectures and seminars, often by visiting research-investigators. One such presenter was a young National Institutes of Health Cardiologist named Harold T. Dodge, MD. [See also "Dedication".]

His lecture described an original x-ray-based method for quantitating the performance of the diseased human heart; measurements including the strength of cardiac muscle and the amount of leakage through an abnormal valve. He used terms I hadn't heard since engineering school: quantitation of flows, pressure profiles, linear fluid velocity, compressive stress, pumping-work and even the heart's mechanical percent-efficiency. All of these measurements were safely made in actual patients and were useful in research and evaluating the need for heart surgery.

Excited at this amalgam of medicine and engineering, I later trained under Dr. Dodge and then served as junior faculty with him at the University of Alabama Medical Center. His scientific philosophy of quantitating everything possible in the circulatory system formed the basis of my own, which served me well through all those years of academic medicine.

So that proved indeed a memorable Sunday School Class for me, even absent hymns and prayers!

Just Like James Bond, Agent 007

One of thousands of truly memorable scenes from the myriad of James Bond movies starting in the 1960s involved his dancing with a beautiful girl (of course!) during Carnival in Rio de Janeiro. But, she was an evil conspirator planning his assassination. He knew this and, "He knew she didn't know he knew." As they waltzed in spectacular style, he gazed lustfully into her lovely eyes, but then saw in their reflection a gun with silencer suddenly protrude through a curtain behind him, aimed directly at his back! He quickly whirled her around as the shot was fired, so that it struck her between the shoulder blades rather than him. As the gunman disappeared, James Bond covered the bullet-hole with his fingers, "danced" her over to a nearby cocktail table and dropped her lifeless body onto a chair. "Do you mind if she rests here awhile? She's so tired, she's just dead," he explained to a fellow-reveler as he departed in pursuit of the villain.

My first rotation as Junior Medical Resident (meaning one year as an MD) was on the Neurology Service at the University of Washington's Harborview Hospital. It was a charity institution, not far from Seattle's famed "Skid Row," so named for the past location where freshly-cut logs were skidded into and out of Puget Sound for transport, as part of the booming timber industry. It was a rough area and at the time home to numerous bums, derelicts and low-lifers; our patient population often reflected this scene. My first neurology admission was a young powerfully-built male, found unconscious and unidentified in an alley. I remember totally puzzling for a diagnosis and phoning the out-going Chief Resident in Neurology at home that night; he had just returned from a party celebrating his completion of training. "I can't understand it – no sign of trauma or drugs, exam otherwise normal, occasional non-purposeful movement, labs okay – like asleep but won't wake up."

"Observe him carefully through the night," he advised, "He'll declare himself. Sounds like a good case for the new Chief Resident in the morning."

The patient's condition remained unchanged.

Next morning I presented the case verbally to our new Neurology Chief Resident during preliminary rounds, prior to formal rounds with our attending neurologist.

"Hmmm," was his thoughtful, scholarly response.

We then proceeded to a bedside neurological examination, the patient reclining "asleep" and partially covered with a sheet. A portion of the exam is called a "Babinski-response", wherein the examiner strokes the bare foot-sole in a carefully prescribed manner with a slightly sharp object, often a house key. The type of toe movement in reaction can give a clue about the condition of certain portions of the central nervous system. The key-stroke is transiently uncomfortable to the patient, though not truly painful.

I stood close to the patient's right side, about waist level, while the Chief stood at the foot of the bed and tested the sole of the patient's right foot for the Babinski-response. After a pause, he said softly, "Baxley, step back about six inches away from the bed."

Now when the Chief Resident says, "Step back," you step back without question. So I stepped back six inches away from the bed.

He then proceeded to stroke the patient's left sole to observe the toe-response.

With lightning speed and in one coordinated move, the patient opened his eyes, sat bolt upright in bed and swung a right-fist powerfully toward my head, just barely grazing, not quite touching, my chin. If I had been six inches closer, I might well have suffered a broken jaw or lost teeth!

It took a number of us to restrain him until a sedative could be injected. Later after the scene finally quieted, I was able to ask, "How on earth did you know to warn me about that?"

"When I stroked his right-sole, I saw one eyelid flutter ever-so-slightly, so I knew he was faking. I suspected violence might follow another uncomfortable stimulus."

So that new Chief Resident in Neurology and this beginning First Year Medical Resident were off to a roaring start!

Sad // A Doctor Matures (-- Somewhat)

I have mixed feelings about the sport of boxing; watching a bout is engrossing, with something elemental, primitive, even compelling about two humans simply fighting viciously in contest. But as a doctor, I wince at repeated head-trauma, knowing that the central nervous system, particularly the brain, to be among the most fragile of human organs. (The eyes would likewise be included, and males might shout, "Testicles also!" But "tenderness" or "pain-sensitivity" is different from "life-altering-injury-vulnerability".) Nature shields the brain nicely within the near-spherical skull. This soft organ also floats in a liquid bath as a further shock- absorbing system. Yet repeated trauma from head-punches can cause minor capillary-bleeding diffusely, similar to bruising elsewhere. But in this fragile organ, such scattered microscopic injury can cause scarring which may disrupt vital neurologic structures and hence function. This in turn can produce a variety of permanent motor (movement) disabilities or other nervous-system dysfunction. Often the result is severe tremor, speech difficulty and muscular incoordination; "punch-drunk" is an appropriate time-honored lay term.

Harborview Hospital in Seattle, Washington, a charity institution and part of the University of Washington system, provided excellent training-grounds for 1960's post-graduate medical education. Electively admitted to its Neurology Service, where I was Medical Resident, was a twenty-nine year old black male. "Diagnosis: Multiple neurologic problems," read the entry sheet. "Occupation: Former prize-fighter. Marital status: single. Home phone: none. Home address: none. Emergency family contacts: none. Personal belongings: Few, arriving with patient. Other information re: patient admission: None."

He was still a relatively handsome fellow, trim and somewhat muscular; alert and smiling. But he exhibited obvious major disabilities: severe intention tremor (i.e., subsiding with rest), marked incoordination precluding walking unassisted and preventing such routine activities as writing and self-feeding. Importantly he had retained bowel and bladder control as well as total-body sensation. Frontal-lobe function (thinking, memory, emotion) was intact. He spoke haltingly but with normal content. Eyes were bright and his demeanor reflected apparent mature acceptance of a permanently-altered physical status.

A large, maybe two-foot square, scrapbook was seemingly his sole possession, and he enthusiastically perused it, haltingly, with any passer-by or available hospital employee (he had no visitors), "pointing" as best he could and "explaining", irregularly, each photograph, letter, newspaper-magazine-or-program article, memento, or souvenir. Attempting to share his past with others seemed his major life-goal.

In his early twenties he had been a promising middle-weight contender for the championship. According to his scrapbook, for years he fought "number-ones" and other highly-ranked boxers. "This kid can really take it as well as hand it out!" Pictures of him at famous restaurants and celebrity functions adorned page after page. A pink Cadillac convertible complete with pretty girlfriend was there; he always beautifully coiffed and dressed, beaming.

Trouble had started as a minor episodic right-hand tremor. Medical tests followed and a rapid devolutionary-spiral ensued, harming all aspects of his life. Gone were the fights, money, glory, fame, and a happy future; instead, a quick fade-out on all fronts.

There was little our neurology team could do other than confirm the diagnosis and arrange for custodial care.

The foremost requisite of any practicing physician is possession of a complete scientific knowledge of her-or-his field of medical endeavor; without this factual basis, the doctor does a terrible disservice to the innocent, trusting patient. However, following closely behind "smarts" is compassion, plus simple common sense. These three elements must be balanced, particularly for physicians attending the severely ill or injured; one must possess feelings for the suffering fellow-human but also avoid becoming so enmeshed in them that scientific thinking is clouded: a certain degree of emotional distance is required between doctor and patient,- not too little nor too much. And "common sense" is a difficult term to define, though most have an awarenesss of its meaning.

I spent worried hours resolving these kinds of emotions after working with this sad case; but I did resolve them, finally realizing the balance of these three doctor-requisites. Later as an academic, I often observed these same types of personal struggles in medical students and young doctors-in-training. But we all either have to resolve them, or as some do, steer oneself permanently into a more tepid corner of the medical realm.

FACULTY YEARS

Close Calls

The Heart's Function Curve

One of the countless marvels of our heart's pumping action is called the "Frank-Starling Curve," named after its 1918 discoverers Otto Frank and Ernest Starling. This curve describes mathematically how the heart's muscular contraction partially empties itself with each beat, the amount ejected depending upon how full it becomes between beats. (This in contrast to our biceps and triceps – "skeletal muscle.") Stated another way, the more the heart is filled and stretched-out between beats, the stronger the contraction. This self-regulating feature helps maintain our circulation nicely through a variety of bodily situations, from high-flow requirements (a one-mile race!) to "idling" when we sleep.

But this characteristic works only up to a point.

If the heart is distended too far, the muscle overstretched, particularly if weakened or blood-starved, it progressively empties itself less with each beat: the dreaded "descending limb of the curve". The result, if uncorrected, is a rapid devolutionary spiral of pathophysiology: progressive cardiac swelling, less output per beat, circulatory failure, shock and death.

Medical students learn this principle in detail; MDs use it daily in prescribing fluids and medications for severely ill patients such as those in intensive care units.

Anyone who has learned emergency treatment techniques, or has even watched medical-drama TV, knows what "CPR" is: cardio-pulmonary-resuscitation. It involves mouth-to-mouth ventilation and regular chest (i.e., external cardiac) compressions. On occasion this procedure can save a life during cardiac arrest. Most often this extreme measure is performed in settings of severe cardiac rhythm disturbances, until such can be corrected and circulation restored.

But not always.

By the 1990s coronary balloon angioplasty had advanced to the point of correcting a patient's numerous blockages in multiple vessels, all during one procedure. My particular interest at the time was the very sickest patients; those turned down for surgery, with weak hearts and other-organ disease – "their last chance."

One such had his procedure utilizing general anesthesia, an anesthetist keeping him nicely asleep and mechanically ventilated. This added step was uncommon, routine angioplasties done with patient awake, local numbing over the femoral (groin) artery only. But I preferred this feature in high-risk settings: more complete blood-oxygenation, with the work of breathing temporarily shifted off of the patient.

His angioplasty was going well up until treatment of the final blockage: a large important artery. It required repeated brief dilations, each causing momentary loss of blood flow downstream to the heart muscle, resulting in fall of blood pressure and rise in filling pressure (measure of the heart's distention); however, his recoveries had all occurred quickly.

But with the final balloon inflation, by necessity prolonged, there was no quick recovery of vital parameters. Instead, with each heartbeat all measures slowly worsened.

The entire team stared at the monitors, transfixed. We all *knew*.

My mind raced: "He's slid onto the dreaded descending limb of Starling's curve! What to do or add? He's already optimally medicated, best heart rate and rhythm, mechanically ventilated by the anesthetist, not enough time to insert a temporary circulatory pump-assist device." (My later simile: "This patient was like a person, dizzy, standing at the very edge of a high cliff, with the wind blowing hard – in the wrong direction!")

Then Johnnie Knobloch, one of our superb scrub-technologists, "Sir, should I give his heart just a little help?"

"Yes."

In a flash, he pushed aside the x-ray equipment, lowered the table, positioned himself adjacent to the patient's left chest, and watching the monitor carefully, began external cardiac chest compressions – gently, not enough to cause chest-wall or cardiac trauma (which can easily occur) – in total synchrony with the heart's own weak contractions as shown on the monitor.

Total silence except for ventilation-wheezing and the monitor's bleeps.

No movement anywhere in the room except the gentle synchronous chest compressions, each helping slightly, the heart's output every beat.

I envisioned the mathematics involved, as the overstretched cardiac muscle gradually crept back up the function-curve and over to its ascending, normal portion.

All eyes glued on the monitors.

Slowly, slowly, arterial pressure bottomed out and began to rise; filling pressure (an indicator of cardiac distension) peaked and started to fall; oxygenation levels climbed.

Three days later the patient was discharged home and walked out of the hospital.

Thanks, Drs. Frank and Starling! (and tech Johnnie Knobloch)

Conference Time

In all teaching hospitals, conferences of various forms and shapes are held regularly for instruction at every professional level – sharing of experiences; in-depth subject reviews; and demonstrations of new and developing technologies and procedures. The following describes a memorable Cardiac Catheterization Conference held at Birmingham's University Hospital in 1990 [with lay-explanations of medical terms where needed.] This weekly meeting reviewed cases of a diagnostic test wherein thin tubes are advanced through blood vessels into the heart for measurements and for angiograms [black-and-white x-ray movies with dye injections, particularly of coronary arteries]. A further step may be taken in selected cases: coronary angioplasty. Here a tiny balloon is fed across a blockage, inflated to correct it, and then withdrawn – all this under local anesthesia and mild sedation, the patient awake with minimal discomfort. Such conferences are attended by all interested medical personnel; faculty physicians and surgeons, cardiology fellows [MDs learning the specialty] residents, students, nurses, technologists and others. [Sadly, because medical-malpractice lawsuits have become so common and such a problem for doctors and hospitals, even case-conferences may be effected: honest discussion may reveal the possibility that a different clinical choice might have led to a happier outcome. Thus some institutions have adopted the rule of requiring a licensed defense lawyer present at all conferences. In this way, relevant clinical material and discussions are protected by attorney-client privilege. Unfortunately this practice adds cost and hampers a valuable learning tool.]

This particular week was my turn as Staff Cardiologist to preside.

(Narrator)

"Our case today is a forty-year old female with exertional chest pain, positive exercise test, and diagnostic angiography showing an isolated severe narrowing in the anterior descending coronary artery [major vessel in the front of the heart]. Interestingly at this young age and gender, she had only a positive family history with no additional risk factors, a non-smoker. She was well otherwise and had been referred for balloon angioplasty."

(Narrator then projects the coronary angiogram [black-and-white movie x-ray] onto the screen before the attendees.)

"Here is our preliminary picture of the anterior artery, taken just before the planned balloon. There is the obvious severe narrowing, our 'target lesion.'" (Points with laser-light.) "But do you see anything else? Look carefully". (Re-plays the film slowly.) "Now here is the image before any dye comes through, and – here now – is the image after it has flushed on by. Dr. ___ (Cardiology Fellow), do you see anything additional of note?"

(Fellow)

(He studies the angiogram closely.) "Yes, look, a little speck of dye remains up there in the main left artery, doesn't flush on through." [The left main coronary artery supplies almost all of the heart muscle, giving rise to the anterior artery and others.]

(Narrator)

"What do you think that is?"

(Fellow)

"Oh, I'm worried the catheter-tip has caused a small trauma to the vessel, maybe loosened a small cholesterol-plaque."

(Narrator)

"Exactly! Worrisome. Why?"

(Fellow)

"That irregularity could cause a sudden blood-clot to form, acutely blocking flow to most of the heart – catastrophic!"

(Narrator)

"Right. So we were very worried. What to do? We reviewed our options: send her at once to by-pass surgery; cancel the procedure; or wait awhile and watch. She appeared fine, stable, felt well. So we waited fifteen minutes and repeated the dye injection and x-ray. No change, the little spot still there but no clot or progression. We decided to proceed with angioplasty of the target lesion. That took about thirty minutes with excellent results." (Shows angiogram with final outcome, the target-narrowing now normal.) "Note the little spot still there, no change. So we terminated the procedure, leaving the little sheath in the femoral artery, capped off until the blood-thinner wore away, then we'd plan to remove that also, per protocol. I went up to the control room and began completing my paperwork. But then, 'Doctor, come back! Problem!' I hurriedly returned to the patient – she was now in severe chest pain, monitors showed blood pressure had dropped to sixty, heart rate up to one-thirty with frequent premature beats [an ominous sign portending cardiac arrest], EKG showing severe ischemia [poor cardiac blood supply]! Dr. __ (Fellow), what has happened?"

(Fellow)

"Oh, wow, I'm fearful that 'little spot' has suddenly formed a clot blocking the left main artery!"

(Narrator)

"Exactly. So we quickly replaced our catheter and re-x-rayed." (Shows angiogram now confirming total blockage.) "The patient is still conscious but deathly pale, severe perspiration. She warns ominously, 'Doctor, I think I'm going to die.' So what to do now? Note her husband and two kids out in the waiting room."

(Fellow)

"Get help, quick!"

(Narrator)

"We called other staff to run here, not walk, contacted the cardiac surgeon on call and advised emergent OR set-up. In addition, we were able to place a small catheter with multiple side-holes, appropriately called a "bail-out device," across the clot, to allow restoration of some blood flow, resulting in improvement in all parameters, but this might well be only temporary. The whole thing could clot again at any moment!

We placed an intra-aortic balloon pump [temporary circulatory-assist device] via the opposite femoral artery as the surgeon arrived and made a quick assessment.

Now I don't want to be overly dramatic at a scientific conference, but the simple fact is that Dr. ___ saved this young woman's life. Sir, tell us about the surgical procedure."

(Dr. __)
(Describes in detail the successful emergency coronary by-pass operation with three-month follow-up evaluation.)

(Narrator)
"Thank you. Obviously big lessons for all of us to learn right here. Remember, this rare complication occurred during the diagnostic catheterization portion of the procedure, not the balloon-angioplasty, which is usually considered more risky. In all my years on staff, I have only seen this particular complication once before, and that concluded fatally before we could rescue him. Catheter manufacturers literally spend millions of dollars trying to make the safest products, but accidents happen.

So you Cardiology Fellows who complete your training and go out into practice doing these diagnostic procedures need to be totally prepared for all complications. When arriving at a new hospital, rehearse, repeatedly, every potential problem with your team; hone your skills with balloon-pump use; and get to know well your friendly heart surgeons.

This concludes our meeting today, but remember to keep eyes and ears open for good teaching cases to use in future conferences."

"Wait -- Who Was That Masked Woman?"

On a particular Saturday afternoon in the early1990's I was staff interventional-cardiologist on call at Birmingham's University Hospital, which means being available for any emergency coronary-balloon angioplasty treatment on patients with stuttering or full-fledged acute heart attacks.

(As pre-amble to recounting this particular drama, a word of medical equipment-description is necessary. Our cardiac procedure-room utilized a complex variety of radiology imaging technologies for visualizing and correcting coronary-artery blockages. Initially the patient would be placed on a table resembling a short, wide diving board, anchored at one end only, to allow free movement of x-ray equipment for optimal viewing angles, different for each individual. Most tables had body-weight limits of about three hundred pounds; ours however could safely support such larger individuals. For this reason we were occasionally referred extra-heavy patients for procedures, in this particular case emergently.)

I was advised of the impending helicopter-arrival of a three-hundred pound male with heart attack in progress. A few minutes later he was wheeled into our procedure room and placed (with difficulty) onto the table, appearing physiologically stable, though still in some pain and distress. He was large-framed and muscular and obese! Because speedy treatment is essential to minimize damage during heart-attacks, we rapidly proceeded to introduce catheters into the vascular system, planning quick x-ray images of the coronary arteries. The results would then reveal the best emergent treatment: medication, open-heart surgery or balloon angioplasty. However, prior to imaging, he abruptly developed ventricular fibrillation (a form of cardiac arrest sometimes complicating heart attacks). Blood pressure plummeted, he became unconscious, and initially our quick electrical counter-shocks across the chest were to no avail in re-starting the heart, partly because of his huge size. Then to compound the problem, he developed a grand-mal epileptic convulsion secondary to the low brain blood flow – an "anoxic seizure." This in turn caused total-body muscle spasm with over-all continuous violent jerking and shaking, threatening to hurl him off of the table onto the floor; and then he stopped breathing! He was rapidly becoming cyanotic (bluish-colored) from lack of oxygen and circulation. We struggled to apply external chest compressions as a form of cardiac massage; to mask-ventilate him; and to intubate his trachea (place a breathing tube orally into the windpipe) – all procedures failing because of his mammoth size, violent tremors and total-body muscle rigor. If we were unable to establish ventilation and circulation quickly, he would die. This was emergency in the extreme! We had already called for Anesthesiology back-up assistance with the pulmonary problem: "CODE BLUE! STAT! STAT! (NOW! NOW!)" About a minute later a nurse-anesthetist raced into the room. She was small in stature (probably ninety pounds, in my later retrospective review), dressed in standard scrub clothes with cap and mask and a surgical gown open in front, which flowed after her like a cape. ("A great green bird swooped into our room," was my subsequent metaphor.) She carried her small tool-box and laryngoscope (lighted tool used for intubating the windpipe). Within seconds she analyzed the situation, administered muscle-relaxant medication to the patient, calming his violent tremors and muscle-spasms, and was then able to flex his bull-like neck back into a more favorable position, pry open his massive jaws, intubate him and begin hand-pumping pure oxygen into his lungs. In the meantime we had restored cardiac function with a combination of cross-chest electrical counter-shock of the highest possible power setting, medication injected through the catheters directly into the heart, and a temporary mechanical circulatory-assist device (intra-aortic balloon pump) positioned via the femoral artery.

Arterial pressure slowly rose and cyanosis gradually abated; he "pinked-up," as we called it. Now significantly improved, he was at least no longer "hanging onto a cliff by his finger-nails."

The nurse-anesthetist proceeded to connect his breathing tube to a mechanical ventilator and to fine-tune its adjustments for optimal blood-gas exchange. When satisfied that all was in order, she transferred her responsibilities over to our cardiac team, wrote her note in the patient's chart and departed the room.

We continued on by imaging the coronary arteries, and with balloon angioplasty, cleared the blockage causing the heart attack, propping it open with a stent. That completed, medication and fluid levels now optimal, we loaded his massive hulk onto a gurney with some difficulty, and pushed him plus multiple accoutrements (intra-venous fluids with medications, monitors, ventilation set-up, circulatory-assist-pump, etc.) with more difficulty, into the coronary care unit to complete his post heart-attack recovery.

After he was "tucked in" (our standard phrase) and under the care of unit-staff, finally I could exhale and breathe a sigh of relief.

I was anxious to look back through the patient's chart to find the name of that valiant nurse-anesthetist (Florence Nightingale? Sakajawea? Joan-of-Arc?) – but her signature was scrawled and unreadable!

Next day I wrote a letter of praise to our Chief of Anesthesiology asking who she was, to permit personal thanks. But he wrote back a curt note stating that a number of staff were on duty throughout the hospital system that day and he didn't know which one she was.

So on a sleepy Saturday afternoon, while most of the local citizenry was at a ball-game or doing chores or drinking beer, an anonymous ninety-pound nurse-anesthetist, performing brilliantly against the harshest of adversity, "with only seconds left to play," had literally snatched the three-hundred pound man from the very jaws of death!

"Politically Incorrect"

Often the most irksome, problematic, and time-consuming tasks for doctors are not medical at all, but rather legal/clerical/ethical/social/financial/educational/political etc., etc.!

The number of ways infection can enter our bloodstream, "septicemia," is endless. Eighteenth and nineteenth century romantic poets liked the theme of the young beauty who pricked her finger on a rose-thorn, causing infection and eventual death in the arms of her weeping lover, she softly lamenting,

> "My life doth ebb,
> And soon 'twill close.
> But remember our love so sweet,
> When the dew lies on the rose."

Okay, so I made that one up, but it does typify the style and sentiment of that flowery era of poetry. The traditional description of such an infection was, "It causes a red streak to slowly creep up your arm. When it reaches your heart, you die." There is an element of truth to this dire warning: what was described defines "septic phlebitis", a progressive infection with secondary blood-clotting inside a major vein, usually caused by some staphylococcus or streptococcus bacterium, common organisms on our skin, gaining entrance through a cut or other injury. Untreated, it actually can cause septic shock and death.

Other possible modes of entry include a miniscule injection directly into our small blood-capillaries: recall that malaria, fatal to many each year even now in underdeveloped locales, enters us through a mosquito's "proboscis" (tiny snout), almost too small to be seen by the naked eye.

Medical workers can be exposed to blood-transmitted disease, particularly hepatitis, by a small skin-scratch in the laboratory, for instance. And AIDS can be contacted by blood or body fluid from a diseased patient.

Sometimes, though rarely, it becomes necessary, even ethical, to make a false statement if, after careful consideration, the situation demands it: thus the famed Italian renaissance scientist Galileo Galilei (1564-1642), after careful measurements, correctly detailed the movements of planets, including our earth, in orbits around the sun. But stating publicly that the earth was not the center of the universe contradicted Roman Catholic doctrine at the time. So appearing before the Pope in Rome during the brutal Spanish Inquisition, Galileo was advised, under threat of bodily harm, to recant his findings in astronomy.

He did so, speaking clearly.

But legend has it that he then muttered under his breath, "Nevertheless it is so."

In the 1990s, we doctors were instructed by Hospital Management not to treat AIDS patients any differently from others, "So as not to embarrass or discriminate against them." No special precautions were to be followed in handling devices such as needles or vascular catheters which had been in their bloodstream during balloon angioplasty: "All patients are to be treated alike."

Totally impractical and downright dangerous!

So on a particular day sometime thereafter, a coronary angioplasty was scheduled on a patient of mine who also had AIDS.

Before starting the angioplasty, I called together the team -- interventional fellow (cardiologist learning the sub-specialty of balloons), medical student, circulating nurse, scrub-technologist and recording-tech -- and instructed thusly, "I may get sent to jail for telling you-all this, but our patient here has AIDS. Be particularly careful of his blood on instruments, needles, catheters, sponges, drapes, etc. and use caution in clean-up afterward. Remember the potential danger to your own health in handling anything with AIDS blood on it." [One team member, noted for his quick wit, then asked, "Sir, I've heard that the best way to avoid AIDS is to always use a condom. Should I go put one on now?"]

50

The procedure and clean-up went smoothly.
I wasn't sent to jail but was chided, "Don't do it again."

"Okay, I won't." But then I was heard to mumble something unintelligible under my breath: "But I will, if needed to protect our workers."

Thanks, Galileo!

"But, Sometimes It's the Other Way Around – "

Cardiac arrest is usually one of two types: the first is "heart block," wherein the upper chambers function normally, but the rhythmic electrical impulse, which originates there and starts each beat, fails to reach the lower pumping chambers. The second type is "ventricular fibrillation"; here the muscle simply quivers, rather than effecting a coordinated contraction. The first type can be treated with pacemakers or medication, the second with electrical countershock to the bare chest. (Medical-TV dramas regularly demonstrate these techniques, mixed in with incredible plot-lines, physical violence, weird characters, stormy emotions, sex, background turmoil, dysfunctional families, personal conflicts, etc., etc.!)

We all have heard the refrain, "Oh, how sad! He was perfectly healthy, in the prime of life, but just fell over dead from a sudden heart attack." Often the adjective used, even by physicians, is a *massive* heart attack. But it may not have been large in terms of size, but rather strategically located within the heart, to trigger one of these two types of potentially fatal cardiac arrest.

All developed countries now have efficient rapid-response medical teams, those "siren-screeching, light-blinding, traffic-stopping EMTs," who can diagnose and treat, at least temporarily, these forms of cardiac arrest (if they get there in time). Such teams are to be lauded and have been proven to increase survival and other measures of happy outcomes from heart attacks and from almost all types of people-emergencies.

But with every form of progress, there seems a down-side: in spite of best efforts by all involved, the unconscious victim may have been deprived of circulation just long enough to suffer brain damage but not to die. So one of the most pressing medical-ethical questions wrought by today's science is, "When do you stop keeping a human alive?" There is no simple answer to this; indeed there may be no answer whatsoever: family wishes, religion, money, hospital resources, science, common sense and multiple other concerns often conflict. Usually, as revealed by news reporters, this problem involves a patient late post head-injury or after an interval of inadequate circulation, such as following a resuscitation. The victim may be termed "in a vegetative state," on life support including mechanical ventilation. Fights may arise among some family members who claim hope ("Look! She seems to be smiling!"), and others more practical ("It's been months with no progress.") Medical testing may not solve the problem either: "The EEG [electro-encephalogram, or brain-wave-test] was inconclusive." And hospital managers worry about a prolonged financial burden. Such a dilemma can produce media frenzy, and it may even reach judicial or national political levels: "The family envisions recovery!"

Often it's a lone family member who has neglected for decades his-or-her relative (now the patient), and feeling subconscious guilt, races to the scene, loudly demanding that "everything possible be done!" When others are finally so convinced, said relative, guilt now assuaged, conveniently departs the chaotic scene to pursue more pleasant activities elsewhere.

But sometimes it's the other way around.

As on-call staff cardiologist one particular day, I admitted a middle-age male heart attack victim brought by ambulance to our Emergency Room. He had been found unconscious, then electrically defibrillated "in the field," as it is termed. Circulation was now adequate though he was still unconscious, requiring mechanical ventilation. After he was settled into our coronary care unit, we instituted standard evaluation-treatment protocols, which were carefully written and frequently updated to ensure the best possible chance of recovery for such patients.

I then asked his nurse, "Are there any family members I can meet with?"

I didn't have to wait for an answer.

A young woman came racing into the room, screaming and waiving a folded piece of paper, "WHAT IS THE MEANING OF THIS? WHY IS MY FATHER ON A VENTILATOR? I DEMAND HE BE TAKEN OFF AT ONCE!"

Whenever I could get a word in side-wise, I tried to explain the situation:

"He's had a heart attack."

"He'll die right now if we take him off."

"Yes, there is the chance of permanent brain damage, but there's also the possibility of full recovery – only time will tell. We'll keep you fully informed."

That didn't slow her: "YOU TAKE THAT OFF RIGHT NOW! I KNOW WHAT YOU DOCTORS DO – YOU KEEP PATIENTS ALIVE FOREVER ON VENTILATORS SO YOU CAN COLLECT YOUR FEES!"

"Ethically I can't do that. There's a reasonable chance he can come off of it later."

She waved her folded piece of paper.

"DO YOU SEE THIS DOCUMENT? IT IS HIS ADVANCE-DIRECTIVE! IT IS SIGNED; IT IS WITNESSED; IT IS NOTARIZED; IT IS REGISTERED AND IT SAYS 'NO VENTILATORS!"

She was causing such a commotion and disturbing other patients that I was on the verge of calling Hospital Security. But then she stomped her foot and, departing, shouted, "I'M GOING STRAIGHT TO MY LAWYER – WHEN HE GETS THROUGH WITH YOU, YOU'LL BE SORRY YOU EVER BECAME A DOCTOR!"

Weaning a patient from mechanical ventilation involves following a carefully prescribed procedure, which may or may not succeed: The percent of oxygen used, the strength and frequency of the "push," and the amount of sedation to the patient are all slowly decreased while carefully monitoring parameters of vital function, particularly tissue oxygenation. If all goes well the machine is removed but the breathing-tube left in place awhile in case needed quickly. Finally it too is withdrawn: "extubation."

The patient was successfully weaned and extubated on day two. Shortly following this was one of those "Happy Hospital Moments": as doctors and nurses stood around the bed, he suddenly opened his eyes, stared about the room and at us wildly, and then with a classic cliché straight out of medical TV dramas, shouted, "WHERE THE (bleep) AM I?"

Smiles and quiet applause erupted from the staff present.

He made a nice early post-heart attack recovery and was discharged home to a rehabilitation program.

I never heard from any lawyer nor was I verbally assaulted further by the daughter, who remained sullen thereafter, in the background. I didn't gloat over this case-handling nor feel smug about it – I simply did what any ethical MD would have done, and I'm sure it would have withstood legal challenge. Nor did I harbor ill will toward the daughter; becoming irrational during personal tragedy seems a human trait we doctors must understand and accommodate.

I was simply glad the case concluded happily.

Not all do.

Death (Part Two -- The Faculty Years)

[It was an old, foreign, black-and-white war film, maybe Russian. The scene was a desolate, tree-less swamp with overcast sky. An isolated, nondescript soldier plods through it, carrying on his shoulders a comrade, either wounded or dead. Total silence except for the regular "slosh, slosh" as he walks slowly along; nothing in the background but empty horizon.

This scene continues unchanging for awhile.

Then a single gunshot rings out, momentarily breaking the silence.

The soldier plods on, bearing his burden.

"Slosh, slosh."

The camera now slowly shifts its focus onto the horizon, away from the soldier.

"Slosh, slosh."

The horizon gradually tilts at an angle, then snaps back straight again. After a moment, it tilts slightly to the other side and remains there. Awhile later the horizon begins to rotate slowly, as if viewed from a barely-moving carousel, then speeding up slightly. The camera almost imperceptibly shifts upward onto the sky, to the sun, and both begin to darken as the image continues to rotate. The "slosh, slosh" slows and finally stops.

The entire image of sun and sky, after a few more moments, becomes totally black.

Any medical doctor would recognize this film-sequence as showing a fatal internal hemorrhage caused by the bullet, probably small caliber and non-expansive, tearing an artery or large vein, likely within the abdomen.

But knowing this pathophysiology in no way diminishes the feeling of pathos and poignancy engendered by viewing this scene – indeed, such knowledge enhances it.]

Early Graduation

Customarily in university hospitals, a junior member of the ward team evaluates each electively-admitted patient first. (In private-practice settings, this task is usually performed by a nurse or physician-assistant.) After reviewing the medical history and laboratory data, he or she performs a physical examination. Later the information is summarized verbally to the team. This junior member may be a medical student, intern or resident, and occasionally the remaining team may be only an attending staff physician such as myself.

On this particular occasion a senior student was my only available team member, the others out on more urgent business. He was a big, athletic, jovial fellow – smart and hard-working, with the wonderful talent of joking with patients to put them at ease.

[This phrase, "joking *with* patients" bears further comment: it is totally opposite to the terrible act of "laughing *at* a patient." I, as all health professionals, have always known this difference and acted accordingly, out of respect for the sick.

Except once.

I was sitting on an examining table behind a female clinic-admission, preparing to check her breathing with my stethoscope. She then advised me something further of her symptoms, a detail of which I found ludicrous. She glanced over her shoulder and saw me silently laughing at her, and she began to cry.

She was ill and had come to me, a doctor, for help, and I had laughed at her.

The only defense I can offer is that just arriving in Saudi Arabia, I was totally disoriented in all spheres. Though this case concluded happily from a medical standpoint, nevertheless it remains an inexcusable professional-ethical transgression on my part.]

Popular with ward staff and patients alike, he would be a doctor soon and a good one.

After performing the initial evaluation on a new female admission, he summarized the clinical data to me just outside her room. As usual, we knocked and entered, intending for me to confirm the findings and to discuss with her our treatment plan.

Once inside, I saw immediately that the woman had been dead for a short time.

There was nothing to be done for the poor lady, so I chose to observe the student. We approached her, he introducing me and explained that I was to check some of his examination - findings. When she did not respond, he assumed she was asleep. He shook her gently, with a little joke about how it wasn't best to nap with the professor present.

Then he too realized that she was dead.

I shall not forget the look on his face as he turned and stared at me, his eyes reflecting the sudden awareness that this fellow human, so vibrantly alive earlier, was now gone, victim of a disease which he struggled so to understand. In a symbolic sense, he did not receive his MD degree some weeks later at graduation, but rather he achieved it that day at his dead patient's bedside.

I have observed this type of emotional scene played over repeatedly with medical students and young doctors, particularly when the technical or scientific aspects of disease initially predominate, but then the drama devolves into the death of an actual person, with all of its humanistic consequences.

Faith

One of the most poignant deaths I ever attended was that of a middle-aged woman in the coronary-care unit of Birmingham's University Hospital where I was Staff Cardiologist. By chance it was also a period of personal turmoil in my own life. The patient knew her medical situation and had requested no late heroic treatment. She was totally lucid and pain free. Since there was no family, as the end approached I sat close and held her hand, the chaplain and her nurse nearby. Her last words were, "Oh, don't worry about me, Doctor – we have just prayed -- I'm not afraid to die. But something in your eyes tells me that you, yourself, are deeply troubled and I'm most concerned about you."

If heaven exists, surely this woman's soul resides there.

"Happy Holidays"

As Staff Interventional Cardiologist, with children grown and gone, I often volunteered for on-call during Christmas, in deference to colleagues with small ones. On one such occasion I received an urgent evening phone call from one of our cardiac surgeons: "Tough problem. Severely ill middle-age male, inoperable, multivessel coronary disease. There's no way we can perform surgery on this man. See if you can help. If not, I doubt he'll make it through the night."

I reviewed his data and met with the family.

"I can't be optimistic, but we'll try."

Coronary angioplasty involves feeding a small deflated balloon over a long thin wire advanced up from the femoral (groin) artery, guided by x-ray. So this requires that the wire first be advanced through the blockage. If said blockage is complete, old and scarred, sometimes we simply can't cross it with the wire, even though made of steel. "Like trying to advance a roto-rooter through a pipe full of rocks."

We tried for hours to cross at least one of this patient's many blockages, using a variety of techniques.

Failure.

All vital parameters dwindled.

Finally I called the team together. "We've tried everything I know. Unless any of you objects or has further ideas, I think we should quit and let him go."

Silence. Reflection. Downcast eyes.

Then one of them, "Sir, I agree, that's the wise choice."

The patient died within minutes.

Then to the family.

Their large group with Chaplain waited in the "quiet room," reserved for such occasions: wife, multiple children, grandchildren, aunts, uncles – all ages, from diapers to walkers.

As soon as I stepped into their world, they all read my face and began to cry.

Then the chaplain, "Let us hold hands and pray for deliverance of his soul."

I join with them.

Driving home alone to my apartment, the first blush of dawn just visible through the freezing rain, I speak aloud to myself in soliloquy, "There must be a happier way to make a living."

"No! Stop it! You're a doctor. You help some people."

"Okay."

Off call now.

Pour some scotch.

Merry Christmas.

SAUDI ARABIA

First Trip: The Seeds Are Planted

It was in the late nineteen-seventies and my personal life was problematic at the time. The middle-east with all of its exotic differences from our standard American culture had always interested me. This, plus a wish for temporary venue change, drove me to save up vacation time and answer a medical newsletter advertisement requesting help at a large teaching hospital in Riyadh. The Saudis, now with big oil-money, were trying to expand and modernize their public medical-care and educational systems at major cities within the kingdom. Thus they sought short-term assistance from western physicians. My application accepted, I made all necessary preparations at the office, and as departure date approached, packed personal belongings into several suitcases and numerous boxes. I vividly recall the night before leaving -- a cold rain falling while I stored the boxes in a rented garage facility. I was with one of the nurses at the time and it was after midnight when finally arriving at her apartment. Up at dawn, some last-minute chores, mailed out a medical research abstract which summarized recent work, with the hope of winning a presentation-invitation at an upcoming scientific meeting; then off to the Birmingham airport. I remember pausing at the bottom of the outside stairway onto the plane, hatless in the cold driving rain, quite exhausted on all fronts, thinking, "If you can make it up those steps, you can leave those personal problems behind and start again with a clean slate."

Finally collapsing into the seat, "I did it."

Then outbound from New York to London, it was one of those huge planes, but oddly there were no other travelers in my portion of the first-class cabin, so my flight-attendant had only me.

She sat close beside me.

We talked and talked -- and talked.

We were both emotionally vulnerable.

She was German, based out of Frankfurt.

She kept pouring martinis.

Of what then transpired I surely am not proud, but it happened and I'll relate it.

I became terribly drunk.

The last thing I remember her saying was, "Don't worry, I'll take care of you." (Only later did I associate that famous line of Tennessee Williams' Blanch Dubois in *Streetcar Named Desire,* "I often rely on the kindness of strangers.")

I vaguely recall being led about, standing in lines half-asleep, sitting somewhere, cat-napping, standing in front of official booths with agents of some sort looking at me, more cat-naps, on and on, then oblivion.

I awakened in a bed, startled, now perfectly lucid, in absolute, total silence and darkness ("Like the inside of a coal-mine at midnight, with the lights off," was my later simile). I had no idea whom I was in bed with or where I was – what city or even country. I had been on my way to Riyadh via London, but then linked up with a German girl who had promised to take care of me. I didn't know what time-zone I was in, or the date – it had been near December's end, so I didn't even know the year.

Groping around, I found a bedside lamp; then groping further, located my passport and money, so I knew I would survive.

I turned off the light and went back to sleep.

Illness is the great equalizer of all humanity, cutting across lines of race, culture, time, age and just about any other variable that categorizes us as people. When Grandmother has chest pains and trouble breathing, the kin take her to whoever or whatever they think can help, whether it be a shaman in ancient India, a modern elegant hospital in Hollywood, USA, or the Saudi Government Hospital in Riyadh. The patient and family arrive with faces reflecting a mixture of fear and hope. The care-provider, doctor or otherwise (if ethical) uses his-or-her knowledge and whatever tools available to treat the sick one as effectively as possible. So I was right at home, even in such a strange land, doing what I have always done professionally as a medical doctor. It was actually a good modern hospital, though the people's customs, dress, language, behavior, habits, and environment were quite different from anything I had ever experienced; however these differences were only a matter of interest and not of importance. People are still basically people, everywhere, in my simple medical philosophy.

Some weeks later in preparing for departure from "The Kingdom" as it is locally called, I planned several stops on the way home; first in Tehran to visit Iranian friends and buy original hand-made silk Persian rugs (Persia the earlier name for Iran, and the tradition of family rugweaving as an art-form continues.)

(Here a brief jump-ahead comment: Tehran at the time was strongly ruled by the USA-friendly Shah Palavi, and the arab region was generally peaceful, in contrast to today. I attended a lavish party given by my doctor friend. Conversing with multiple other guests, (English widely spoken by those educated) a varied group of locals, I recall musing, "There seem three different cultures here: one the pro-western Shah faction, then the leftist group (a young lad just released from jail for criticsizing the Shah), and finally the strict Muslim religious faction. I wonder what the future holds for this country, with such stringent cultural diversity.")

From Tehran I planned to fly on, to drink Spanish wine with colleagues in Madrid; and finally from there to Santo Domingo ("just like Columbus traveled almost five centuries earlier, but a bit faster now") to buy locally-mined amber and for some beach-R&R before home and work. To enter Iran required a visa which could only be obtained in Jedda, the major Saudi Red Sea port. Someone commented to me, "Oh, if you go there, you should snorkel out over that spectacular Red Sea reef north of the city." So a companion and I flew to Jedda, rented a car, obtained the visa, bought camping and snorkeling gear, then headed north. We pitched our tent on a beautiful desolate beach, and early morning next in bright sunshine, with flippers, mask and snorkel, I waded out alone into the totally clear, quiet water. The sandy bottom-slope was gradual, and it was fifty yards or more before deep enough to swim, then another fifty or so before the reef appeared. Cruising out over it, I was at once amazed. The water was as translucent and peaceful as air; the coral forming a sharp, deep cliff parallel to shore – beautiful pink, grey-green, mauve, yellowish and aqua hues, ragged and irregular in form. I thought, "an underwater Grand Canyon!" The sea was alive as brightly-colored fish of all shapes and sizes swam slow or fast, in schools or solo. It was indeed an impressive vista of silent natural beauty, both still and in motion. Because the Saudis are by nature desert-folk, not seamen, fishers, sailors, or divers (in contrast to Egyptians on the other side of the Red Sea), an eerie feeling developed within me that this reef was virgin.

But quickly back to my companion on the beach, for if young local males were to chance upon an unescorted western female in a remote location, the result at best would be cat-calls and epithets; at worst, gang rape.

She was a delightful companion – smart, independent, pretty, with an eye and an ear to the world – a true adventuress. Her job was clerical at the hospital, and soon after we became "friends," her supervisor called her into his office and instructed her to seduce me and then entice me into staying, as the hospital needed doctors! We both absolutely howled at that! But I couldn't stay. My body (literally), soul and heart belonged to Birmingham's University Hospital. Nevertheless, at that time in my life, it did seem appropriate to pause a moment, look around, but then recall those terse poignant lines of American poet Robert Frost: "Yon wood is inviting, dark and deep, but I have promises to keep, and miles to go before I sleep."

Still, she and I had adventures there in the Kingdom. Once while driving over the lace-work of roads, from camel-paths to freeways, that pattern some portions of the desert, through a series of compounding navigational errors, we found ourselves inside the Muslim religion's sacred city of Mecca! An unmarried western couple, -- infidels! -- within that forbidden, heavily guarded, holiest place, strictly off-limits to all but devout followers of the Koran!

We escaped. But that's another story.

So the image of that hauntingly-beautiful Red Sea reef was implanted into my being. It added to my earlier realization that these different foreign-folk present an interesting challenge regarding medical care. Hopefully someday I, a doctor, would return to Saudi Arabia, such a strange-but-intriguing land, to further assist their attempts in this humanitarian endeavor, for a longer stay (and return also as a trained scuba diver).

Second Trip, For a Year!

Life in a – Different/Same – Type Hospital

Oh, Wow! Back again to this strange – but somehow interesting, even enticing, and in some areas actually beautiful, land. And this time granted a leave from my regular work for the entirety of 1983! (Christian calendar, not Muslim with its totally different notation) From my earlier short visit, I knew what to expect and was looking forward to it, even though friends had warned , "You're crazy for going so far away for so long. You'll miss the ol' USA!" However, I'm a wanderer at heart, and during that year I was given considerable off-time and was able to travel Europe, Africa, India, Sri Lanka, Thailand, Nepal, and Pakistan. But wait, I'm getting ahead of my story.

Last trip I had worked in Riyadh, the centrally-located capital metropolis close to the "empty quarter", a huge, well-named desert. This time I chose Taif, a smaller city one-hundred miles inland from the major Red Sea port, Jedda. Important for me, our hospital, Al Hada, was a teaching institution affiliated with Jedda University, with medical students, interns and residents. Additionally Taif lay in one of Saudi's few mountain ranges with high altitude (5400 feet above sea level, a little higher than Denver) and relatively cool climate, nice for this "zany early-morning runner." And the Red Sea was easily accessible!

I was provided a nice apartment near the hospital, shared with an American internist who quickly became a scuba dive-buddy, but I'll relate those tales later. Al Hada Hospital provided interesting work from multiple standpoints: clinical, humanitarian, educational and even investigative (I'd brought along research projects needing work). We treated all patient-levels, male and female, from the Royal Family to the lowliest shop-keepers. [Notice I didn't write "to the poverty-stricken". There is no poverty in Saudi Arabia. The government is a benevolent monarchy in terms of finances. To some groups about the world, this statement constitutes an inconvenient truth.]

One unique advantage provided all practicing physicians world-wide is interacting with locals on a personal, even professionally-intimate level, patients mostly being honest and open and not playing psychological games with their doctors; this leads us to a surprisingly deep understanding of the national culture. Few other professions enjoy this advantage. Of course this benefit also pertains within one's own country and society.

Our hospital staff was constantly engaged in expanding in-patient and clinic facilities and activities. As always I enjoyed working with and teaching medical students, interns and residents, including the few female trainees. Those few dressed modestly, as required of all women in the Kingdom (and men too, for that matter), but were bare-faced in contrast to most others, whose "abayas" cover totally. This gender of physicians would ultimately be restricted to pediatrics, obstetrics-gynecology, or all-female practices. Nevertheless, they were breaking out of the restrictive wife-only tradition and I happily promoted their endeavors and admired their courage.

Any western physician working away from home, elsewhere on the globe, encounters different illnesses and afflictions than we are used to: sometimes less common specific diseases than we Americans experience. For instance some poorer countries have markedly fewer high blood pressure problems, heart attacks and strokes than we – by virtue of their healthier life-styles, diet and possibly heredity.

But our American medical-care system and hygienic habits do protect us such that we doctors can be surprised when working elsewhere. In a cardiology example, chronic rheumatic heart disease with damage to cardiac valves is a late-sequel of infections by streptococci bacteria. Childhood pharyngitis is its most common clinical precursor, but "strep-throat" is rapidly cured by penicillin or other antibiotics. Physicians in our country diagnose and successfully treat this infection such that rheumatic heart disease has become quite uncommon in the US. But elsewhere, as I quickly learned, one best be ever-suspicious of this diagnosis, even in its most rare and bizarre manifestations. The chronic form can be controlled medically in many cases and, if necessary, corrected by heart valve surgery.

[Funny story here: good-quality heart surgery is available in Riyadh and several other Saudi cities, though not at our smaller hospital. However, members of the Royal Family often preferred London. Cardiac surgeons there, like all UK physicians, are salaried members of their National

Health Service, and some of those MDs are not too happy about it and are thus often in a bad mood. But they are permitted to accept outside private referrals. So on occasion I would telephone a London heart surgeon and be answered rather brusquely, "Yeh? Who-zis? Whada-ya-want?"

"This is Dr. Baxley, cardiologist in Saudi Arabia. I have a patient referral for you."

Then -- instant change! "Oh, how nice of you to call, Doctor! And when would the patient like to come? And how many family members? We'll be happy to make all the arrangements, provide elegant quarters and meet the plane with limousines and attendants!"]

Fatal snake-bite is rare in the USA, but not so everywhere. Indeed hundreds if not thousands die annually world-wide from snakes, mostly in tropical or hot wilderness locations.

An American construction-worker on a remote Saudi desert project arose one night and ventured outside of his trailer, barefoot (against rules), to urinate. He felt a pricking sensation on his foot, but paid it no heed, suspecting some type of thorn-scratch. He returned to bed but later that night suffered a grand-mal seizure, became psychotic requiring restraints, and was febrile.

The ability of our life-sustaining blood to circulate freely within our bodies, but then to clot locally when needed at an injury-site, is indeed astounding. Some minute details of this ability even now remain obscure to medical science.

The pit-viper is a poisonous snake that, like many of nature's desert-creatures, remains in holes shielded from the sun by daylight, but then lurks out hungry during the cooler night. Its venom, like that of some other dangerous creatures, causes a disruption of our normal blood-function. The result is small blood-clots in vital body organs, together with diffuse bleeding. (Venom is not alone in producing this deadly result; other insults including severe infection, shock, and extensive trauma can cause it.) Bleeding in the brain, heart, kidneys and elsewhere can lead to a devolutionary spiral terminating fatally.

By the time this patient reached our hospital late-morning, he was in critical condition, violently combative, hallucinating, wide-eyed. He died that evening of multi-organ failure, a shocked and grieving wife flown in at bedside. This death occurred in spite of excellent treatment in our intensive-care unit, plus a British Tropical Medicine Specialist, well versed in snake-bite diagnosis and treatment, as attending physician.

I suppose I handle patient deaths as well as do most doctors, though sometimes I'm not sure, maybe more sensitive and philosophical. This one especially sad, particularly for the wife, now alone in such a strange place, the death sudden, unexpected, so bizarre.

"The marvelous thing is that it's painless," he said. "That's how you know when it starts."

"Is it really?"

"Absolutely. I'm awfully sorry about the odor though. That must bother you."
>   Opening lines, *The Snows of Kilimanjaro,* short story by Ernest Hemingway

Gangrene is an infectious disease of major historical importance, particularly in wartimes. Before the twentieth century its treatment often defined the work of surgeons: amputations -- gruesome work before the development of general anesthesia in the mid-1800's.

Whenever any of our body's tissues are deprived of blood and hence oxygen, changes begin, with loss of function and sometimes, depending on location, the development of pain, nature's warning. If the deprivation is only transient, termed ischemia, the tissue regains function and normality. But if prolonged, the cells die and totally degenerate. Various body-parts exhibit different time-sensitivities before decreased function and finally cell death occurs.

In example, loss of brain blood-flow will cause fainting (cell dysfunction) in only seconds and, within minutes, brain-death. In contrast, bone, with its slow metabolism and sluggish blood flow is much more resilient in this regard (also the reason fractures take months to heal).

Once cell or tissue-death occurs, it becomes susceptible to any nearby, ever hungry bacteria. These in turn multiply and emit toxins which attack and kill surrounding living cells and they may enter the circulating blood, "bacteremia" or "septicemia", so spreading to distant sites; the next step can be septic shock (fall in blood pressure) with multi-organ failure leading to death.

Doctors know all this in detail, and maintaining adequate tissue oxygenation is a daily must in routine patient care. Severe trauma, or even disease in some cases, can cause blood-vessel disruption and death to a large portion, usually the most distal part, of an arm or leg. Claustridia perfringens, one type of common bacteria and a major cause of gangrene, set up shop and trouble begins.

Such infection is characterized by black discoloration of the effected site, with progression proximally (toward the body). It is, as noted by Hemingway, usually surprisingly painless and accompanied by a horrible, distinctive smell. Bubbles may form on the surface and burst ("gas gangrene") as the claustridia digest dead and living debris.

In modern times, gangrene occasionally occurs in the toes of patients with peripheral-vascular disease, "atherosclerosis," blocking blood supply, particularly in diabetics. This may even require amputation. Fatal gangrene is rare, but it does still occur in remote geographical locations.

Admitted to our hospital was an unfortunate middle-aged Saudi Bedouin female who had suffered major leg-trauma far out in the desert, with no emergent medical treatment. The trip to us had been long and arduous, hot and dirty, rough and uncomfortable. By arrival, gangrene had progressed all the way up her thigh into the hip and lower torso, making surgery impossible and antibiotics unsuccessful. The odor was strong and distinctive, sweet and death-like, in spite of our nurses' best attempts with fans, ice and deodorizers. Strangely the woman felt well, as noted in Hemingway's story, chatting noisily with friends and family at bedside.

But she soon lapsed into a fatal coma.

So we, with our specialty-teams and intensive care unit, were unable to save this poor woman.

I took some solace in learning that the Saudi Government was working hard to develop emergency medical-evacuation systems for these Bedouins, these proverbial desert wanderers.

(For a fascinating description of this rapidly-vanishing culture, read "Arabian Sands" by Wilfred Thesiger, Viking Press, 1983.)

I was asked to consult on a member of the Saudi Royal Family hospitalized with fever of unknown origin. (Fevers can be caused by a variety of diseases, malignancies and metabolic or inflammatory disorders for instance, in addition to infections; exact diagnosis in "FUO" can be elusive even to the most persistent physician.)

"Not my specialty but I'm happy to oblige." I wanted to be sure he didn't have bacterial endocarditis, a rare infection of the heart valves, often difficult to diagnose and deadly if not properly treated.

He was a wizened elderly man in bed, speaking perfect English, dark eyes bright. After proper introductions, he lamented to me that as a young prince he could spring straight from the ground onto his bare-back horse – now he wasn't even able to ride (Arabian horses noted for their beauty and strength).

He was neatly covered with a pile of blankets. Nearby against the wall stood a row of attentive, silent male Royal Family members, finely attired in beautiful, gold-trimmed black ankle-length gown-like garments -- thobes -- with traditional bright head-scarves. Each time the patient made the slightest move, they would all rush forward and pull the covers tightly about him, a move motivated by familial caring.

After surveying the situation, I instructed the nurse, "For starters, he doesn't need all those blankets. Remove them except for a single one of light cotton."

So she removed the extra covers.

And his fever soon resolved!

A week later I received a late-evening phone call; "Doctor, please come over to the Hospital Director's Office." [Saudi Arabia, like most desert countries, conducts much business at night to avoid the heat. Shops and businesses remain closed from noon to evening, then reopen until 10:00 PM or so.]

My first thought was, "Oh boy! What trouble am I in now?"

My boss sat at his desk; beside him stood a handsome young Prince, smiling and resplendent in his black gold-trimmed royal attire. After fitting introductions, the Prince stated, "Doctor, we all appreciate your help in treating Grandfather. He's home now and feeling well."

And, in gratitude, he presented me a Rolex watch.*

Sometimes common sense prevails!

*This watch tells another funny story. In 1983, soon after my return to the US from Saudi, my apartment was rifled by a pot-head druggie, multiple valuable items stolen. I thought the Rolex was among them, and I mused, "Ironically this expensive watch was given me in a country with no drugs, no crime, and limited freedom. Then it was stolen in a country with drugs, crime and freedom." But, low and behold, thirty-three years later, in cleaning out old "stuff," there was the watch, working perfectly after its "lengthy hidden sojourn!"

Beautiful Horses (and an Illicit Love Affair)

A free mid-week afternoon coming up, something rather unusual for me. Chatting with one of our American Radiology Technicians, she, "Oh, I'm off, too! Come ride with me from the City Stables. Some really spectacular horses. I'll show you." She was young, slim, friendly, dark-haired (which of course was covered when around local folk); not one whom I would term "beautiful", but attractive, outgoing, talkative.

(I knew just a bit about horses from younger times spent about the scrub desert of west Texas. Arabian steeds are known for beauty and strength – and fast, having been selectively bred for centuries by various wealthy middle-eastern nobles.)

"Sure! Why not?"

The weather nice, a rarity for the region, and our desert terrain from the stables ideal; soft hills, sparse growth, uninhabited.

We rode a pair of beautiful spirited animals she had expertly chosen. A superb rider, her hair now loosed and flowing, she talked on happily about her past in the US and activities now in the Kingdom; it obvious that a major life-theme was love of horses. She described in detail various breeds, their characteristics and health issues, personalities, training, and so on. Her plan was to save most Saudi earnings and, after a few more years' work, to purchase some quality animals after returning home. Family and friends were never mentioned, and no hint of any romantic interests. I thought, "Fascinating. This girl is certainly smart and attractive from multiple aspects, but she seems to lavish all of her affection and interest on horses."

At the end of our desert sojourn with its lengthy conversation, she must have decided to trust me. She then eyed me carefully, and, "Doctor, would you like to have dinner with my friend and me?"

"Sounds good."

Speaking seriously, "But I must warn you: Be very cautious. Do as I do. Be polite but don't ask any questions. And later don't tell anybody – ANYBODY – about this! Do you understand?" She eyed me sternly.

"Of course. I know what you mean." I was well versed in the rules of social behavior in Saudi Arabia, the most strict of Muslim countries. One either follows them or is expelled out on the next airplane; not physically harmed, as some, who have never been there, would have you believe.

(I had learned these rules early-on. My first night there I was called to the hospital Emergency Room to evaluate a woman with chest pain. After examining her and reviewing other clinical data, I reassured her and family, prescribing a mild sedative. Later I was tending to paperwork in the nurses' station. It was rather crowded, with doctors, nurses, techs, secretaries, etc., many chatting away, writing, phoning – the same as in hospitals worldwide. Someone asked me about my patient. I answered, "She's okay, a little anxiety attack." Then, innocently, adding, "I surely understand her, the way they treat women in this country." And, WOW, a sudden total silence in the entire room, all motion stopped! An American RN quickly pulled me into a closet and slammed the door shut.

"You dumb (bleep)!! You'll get your (bleep) kicked out of this country your very first day here!!"

"Wha'd-I-do-wha'd-I-say-I'm-sorry-I'm-sorry – what??"

She proceeded to lecture me on the detailed rules of social behavior in Saudi Arabia.

I never again had a problem with conduct or manners there.)

After tending and stabling our mounts, her hair now once again concealed, she led me to a covered driveway behind late afternoon shadows. Two local males in traditional robe-like dress stood talking nearby. An automobile with darkened windows approached slowly, she covertly pointing to the two men. The car continued on by. Finally the men left. Again the car approached but now stopped. She directed me to enter quickly with her, and we drove off at once. I was introduced to the sole occupant, the driver male, young, handsome, dark-skinned, dressed casually in western attire (as some Arabs do on occasion), speaking perfect English.

Their dwelling was traditional Saudi: small, cozy, sparsely furnished, no wall art excepting a portrait of the King.

We enjoyed a pleasant simple dinner, just the three of us (no alcohol of course).

Our talk was polite, lighthearted, supposedly superficial, but actually revealing to close-listening: they were lovers and this their hideaway, their place of tryst. They made an attractive pair but their relationship had to remain secret, not because either was married but because he was a Saudi-national, Muslim, she western, non-.

Later they carefully returned me to my apartment.

In this short interlude I had grown to like them both and to admire their courage.
.

I have often wondered how this intriguing story, this Arabian *Romeo and Juliet*, concluded. Knowing what I do of Saudi culture and customs plus US-same, from living and practicing medicine (with its unique window into the local citizenry) in both countries, I can't be optimistic. But her love of horses would sustain her through the ensuing emotional trauma.

Scuba-Diving the Red Sea

"Up, up, you lazy bums! It's dive-time!"

I crawl out of some totally weird dream and grope slowly toward partial reality and awareness; then finally, here I am in our small apartment beside Al Hada Hospital in Taif, the Kingdom of Saudi Arabia. I blink; there, inches before my face is John, screeching, "It's nearly five AM! The reef is calling!"

Coffee; then he, Rod, Mark, (my three dive-buddies) and I pile into our American SUV, pre-loaded last night with all needed equipment. We head south-west down the "escarpment," a twenty-mile two-lane series of steep hair-pins leading from over a mile high down to near sea-level. Now eighty-or-so miles per hour over almost empty desert freeways for another seventy minutes, then, "There! There!" (all pointing), the beautiful, quiet, deserted, majestic, blue-green sea explodes into view. No remnants of bed-time lethargy now -- pure excitement/anticipation! After parking some fifty miles south-east of Jedda in the small coastal hamlet, Shoiba, where our dive-boat "Barracuda" sleeps other days, we transfer equipment and make ready. She's twenty-four feet and open, loaded with coolers for our catch, steering wheel amidships and a well-oiled outboard motor. We ease out from shore, then race to a favorite "Twenty Mile Reef" (a guess – few maps and no sea charts in Saudi. It seems to us about that far offshore.) The sun now clears the horizon, and, I swear, it seems to wink, "Good Morning, Divers!"

So other than medical activity, for me the second major face of Saudi Arabia was the Red Sea dive-scene. Absolutely no social life, though fellow-expatriates and I sometimes gathered to watch (censored) VCR movies in our small apartments. This suited me fine – pretty busy. We doctors plus other medical staff worked hard in our hospital six days a week, but the Muslim Sabbath is Friday; Sunday a regular work-day. (No Christian churches allowed in the country, although some individual small groups worshiped privately in their living areas.) So instead of the relief "TGIF" (Thank God it's Friday!) we'd say "TAIT" (Thank Allah it's Thursday!)

So most Fridays were dive-days.

It all started upon my arrival at the hospital, day-one. I inquired about possible Red Sea scuba-folk and was quickly directed to John Cooney, a Registered Nurse from the UK; "Ireland!" he was quick to correct; a ball of fire, multi-talented, and obviously passionate about diving. I had only recently completed my underwater-course and qualification dive in the US, then packed (along with enough personal items for a full year) buoyancy-vest, pressure-regulator, mask and snorkel, to be ready. John invited me, "straightaway to go diving Friday next!" I was introduced to dive-boat *Barracuda* (later to buy a share of her ownership). And then to spear-guns; big, powerful, more like harpoons. John had bought them on a recent Australia trip.

So my first journey out: pure sunshine, a light breeze, placid water, total desolation. We stopped at one of John's favorite reefs, anchored, then over the side – beautiful! Water so clear. Stunning color. A different, silent, idyllic world. Though he always brought his gun, I declined on a first dive. Better to trail him and get acquainted with this new environment before introducing trauma. Over thirty minutes or so John made six shots at nice, medium size (eighteen to twenty-four inch) edible-type fish: amberjack, grouper, redfish, tuna. Six kills.

He sequentially attached them through gills to his "stringer", a metal holder resembling a two-foot long safety pin, tied to a coral spire.

But then on this seventh shot, the spear only nicked the tail of a fast redfish – not a deadly wound but enough to cause a slightly awkward swim-pattern. Then out of nowhere raced a big barracuda, like a small torpedo, not undulating as other fish. ("They have little invisible propellers," explained John later.) In a flash the barracuda bit the red in half, swallowed both and disappeared!*

Such was my introduction to the savage side of the "Beautiful Red Sea."

I was to see more of this side as the year 1983 unfolded.

*See "Illustration Legends" herein for another barracuda tale from John's repertoire.

After two air-tanks and a couple of hours, with several large coolers of iced fish, well over one-hundred pounds, ready for sale to appreciative hospital-folk (John had rigged a scale in the back of his SUV), we looped through Jeddah for miscellaneous supplies and then headed home. (! -- This was now my home.)

[A brief historical interlude here: In the empty desert near the city of Jedda, while travelling back to Taif after that first dive, I was surprised to see from the highway a large old-fashioned railroad steam-locomotive lying there alone on its side; no tracks, signs, or explanatory notations. It was obviously weather-beaten (but not rusted – no rain, ever). Intrigued and later researching, I discovered it was a historic relic, a memento of the famed T. E. Lawrence: "Lawrence of Arabia." A British Army officer in World War I, he had earlier gained a first-hand knowledge of Saudi Arabia, at that time primarily a desert wasteland occupied by various tribes but officially ruled by the Ottoman Empire (meaning for us today: Turkey). Those Turks at the time were important military allies of Germany. The British leadership wisely sent Captain Lawrence to western and northern Saudi as a "lone wolf", an independent operative, to organize those tribes he knew so well against the Turkish Army stationed there. This he did with amazing success, as detailed in his autobiography, *"The Seven Pillars of Wisdom"*, and as revealed in the award-winning 1962 film, *"Lawrence of Arabia"* starring Peter O'Toole. A favorite guerrilla tactic of his was placing explosives on the railroad track in front of an approaching Turkish troop train; then with his pro-British tribesmen hidden close, blow the track just before the train arrived. After the locomotive plus cars derailed, wrecked and rolled over in the desert, Lawrence leading his tribesmen swooped down and massacred all survivors.

So this particular relic had been lying there untouched for sixty-six or so years, a sad and unappreciated memorial to -- how many deaths? – on some fateful day around 1917. I suspect it will lie there in the dry desert for a thousand years more, perhaps on a few rare occasions piquing the interest of a another foreign visitor such as me.

After learning all this, I felt that history had reappeared in this remote location before my very eyes!]

(Now returning to my post-first-dive story:) I was then introduced to the two other divers, just back from foreign travel; Rod (my assigned apartment-mate) and Mark, both American MDs. After unloading the SUV and selling the catch, John, Rod and I chatted in our apartment living room.

John, "Well, Bax, what do you think?"

"I'm at a loss for words – can't even imagine any – stunning sounds too small. But I will tell you, I'd surely like to dive with you guys every possible Friday.

I do have one question, though. Why do you have such a giant anchor and its hawser line? Big enough for a boat two or three times the size of *Barracuda*, with multiple huge knots in the line."

John and Rod exchanged knowing glances and soft smiles.

Then John, "Bax, pour yourself a fresh cup of coffee, have a seat, prop your feet up and we'll explain."

They proceeded to relate a truly amazing, unforgetable tale of courage, strength and determination that had occurred some weeks previously. [A disturbing 2003 movie, "*Open Water*", based on a true incident, was similar to this tale but with a tragic ending. For a diver, the film was very disturbing, particularly the deleted scenes, which can be retrieved on the DVD version.

I could never watch it again.]

Rather than my retelling their story, I have here provided an excerpt from one of Rod's personal Newsletters, which he sent regularly to friends and family from Saudi; this one written soon after the event (with his permission).

Saudi Roddy Newsletter #7
Long Distance Swimathon
OR
"Hey, man, which way to da beach?!"

Our subject today is scuba diving and long distance swimming. "Hmm, interesting," you say, "but how could those two possibly be related?" Just remember, we are dealing with Saudi Roddy here, a strange man in a strange land.

I hadn't been diving for a while and was anxious to get a little fish blood on my new spear. So we hurriedly loaded the boat, navigated the channel, and headed southwest at full throttle, just John and I and the bright blue sky. The weather was close to ideal: a two to three foot swell but very little wind. Such an exhilarating feeling to leave the Saudis all on shore, just the roar and scent of an outboard motor, the wind and sun and salt spray, and freedom! John drove and I navigated, and with one minor course adjustment, I took him right to Grouper Reef [about ten miles out and so named for the abundance of fish].

The first dive was uneventful and we speared a half dozen fish or so. I had my new underwater 8 mm movie camera, and got some good shots of a large manta ray, and some others of John shooting fish. For the second dive we decided to move to the most leeward point of the reef, since we hadn't dived there before. When we anchored we found ourselves just beyond the protection of the reef so that the swell rocked the boat a bit, but it was already after noon, so we hurried into the water, never giving our mooring a second thought. The second dive was even better than the first, as is often the case: once we get some blood circulating in the water, fish in great numbers come to investigate. A four or five foot white tip shark also came and circled 'round and 'round, obliging my camera. By the end of the dive we both had stringers full of fish, so we surfaced satisfied, ready for the thirty-minute ride back to the beach.

Will I ever forget that sensation that overcame me when I surfaced, looked around, and realized that the boat was gone? The only remotely similar feeling I've ever experienced is when I've discovered something stolen: a kind of sinking of the spirit down, down, down. But never before had it threatened my survival. Now it seems kind of funny, but at that moment I felt as if all the good forces in the universe had deserted us. Now we were at least ten miles out with no boat, no food, no water. Slightly frantically, we swam over to the reef in hopes of spotting the boat, but she was nowhere in sight. She must have torn loose from the coral head she was anchored on at the beginning of the dive, and floated southeast at a couple of knots with the current.

So we sat down on the reef and discussed the options, surprisingly rationally. None of the Saudi fishermen come out that far, so staying where we were without drinking water was out of the question. We had people waiting for us on the beach, who would realize that something was amiss that afternoon, and notify the Coast Guard. Now when I say "Coast Guard," the average American will conjure up an image of huge cutters, clean white uniforms, and heroic efficiency. The Shoiba coast guardsmen are my friends, but basically they are somewhat less than awe-inspiring as potential rescuers: I didn't feel like betting my life that they could find two little heads bobbing in the sea, or even sitting up on a reef. I can swim a mile in our pool in about twenty-seven minutes. But John can't swim well without fins. So we decided to keep our scuba-gear on and swim by finning, for two reasons. One is that we have inflatable jackets (called buoyancy compensators, or "B.C.s") as part of our standard gear, so we could stop and inflate them to rest whenever necessary. Secondly, I have a compass on my depth and pressure gauge console, enabling us to head directly where we wanted to go. Navigating by sun or stars may be fine for sailors, but it is pretty difficult for swimmers. And the part of the beach where we launched is very sparsely settled, so if we missed the coast guard station, we would have to walk miles in the heat without water, as all the weekenders would have gone home by the time we anticipated landing.

It was just about 2 p.m. when we started out, heading 65 degrees by the compass. We were hoping to make a mile an hour, more or less, which would get us home in 10 or 12 hours. So we swam 25 minutes, then took a five minute break, then 25 more minutes and so on, and on. Doing an unaccustomed exercise repetitively is uncomfortable, to say the least. Doing it with rubber fins on makes it even less pleasant. I was never bothered much by muscle fatigue, but my feet hurt more than just a little. Have you ever seen skin that has been in salt water for 20 hours? It looks like wet Kleenex, and the slightest trauma leaves a deep abrasion. There wasn't much epidermis left on the pressure points the next day. As I mentioned, swimming in the open sea, out of sight of land, is a very lonesome experience. With your eyes only inches above water level, you can't see more than a few dozen meters in any direction. You try not to think about your pains, or your hunger, or your thirst. You try to forget about the sharks that you know are down there, realizing that the odds are you won't be attacked. Those odds didn't reassure me much about 6 p.m. when I looked down and saw a five foot white tip circling us. Now as scuba divers we are not afraid of these little guys. When we're down at depth, with a loaded spear gun in our hands, we're more than a match for them. But swimming on the surface, and my spear gun back on Grouper Reef: that's a different ball game. Dying fish float to the surface, and anything flopping around up there looks suspiciously like dinner to myopic Mr. Shark.

When diving, we all try to avoid spending time on the surface. But now we had no choice, so I just hoped this guy had eaten a nice lunch, and would realize that we were bigger than he was, and wouldn't try taking a bite out of my butt. He followed us for about 20 minutes, and then was seen no more. Soon thereafter it got dark: maybe there were still sharks down there, but at least I didn't have to look at them!

We managed to maintain our senses of humor, as truthfully, the whole situation was pretty ridiculous: half bad luck, half carelessness. We told stupid jokes, sang off key, and daydreamed about cold soft drinks. I remember thinking that I definitely was not going to give up because that would be a really stupid way to die and I didn't want my family and friends shaking their heads in sad remembrance and muttering to themselves, "What a stupid – he was!"

For me, the worst part of the night wasn't thirst or hunger or fatigue; it was heartburn. I'd had nothing but coffee and a few fig bars for breakfast, and I have a sensitive gastrointestinal tract. About every half hour I would reflux some acid into my esophagus, making me feel like someone just stabbed me in the chest with a jalapeno pepper. Ahh, my kingdom for some Rolaids!

We'd only slept four or five hours the night before because of trouble with the trucks. About 2 a.m., swimming ever northeast, we hit an emotional, mental, and physical nadir. Okay guys, the joke is over now, I quit, you can pick me up now and take me home to my warm, comfortable bed and a gallon of ice water. But quitting isn't even a consideration, is it? What are the chances of someone spotting two heads bobbing in the waves? No, I resigned myself to swimming within hailing distance of the shore, or perhaps right to the shore if my compass calculation was errant.

The wind picked up a bit in the wee hours, and though the water was about 80 degrees, the air became cold: teeth-chattering cold. I'm hungry, I hurt, I'm exhausted, I'm thirstier than I've ever been or hope to ever be again – do I have to be cold, too? Okay Boss, whatever you say. Too tired to keep swimming, but too cold to stop. For half an hour John and I stopped, inflated our buoyancy compensators, and embracing each other to stay warm, tried to sleep. It wasn't exactly stage four deep sleep, but I did manage to mentally drift off to another world, devoid of the physical suffering that this one was serving.
With that 30 minute break we felt a little better, and so pushed on. Before that rest I had been half asleep while swimming, but shortly afterward we ran into some man-o-wars: large stinging jellyfish. I got hit on the left upper arm and left leg, a glancing blow by a tentacle that took my breath away such a sudden piercing pain like a hot knife blade twisting in my flesh. The pain was agonizing for five minutes, intense for 30 and merely bothersome after that. It did keep me wide awake while I swam, though.

Through the night we could see lights on shore, so we knew we were going in the right direction. But we had no way of judging how far away they were, so couldn't tell how much progress we were making. I was just hoping that the morning light wouldn't reveal that we were still five miles away, as I wasn't in the mood for any discouragement. Finally around six the first rays of a brilliant sunrise ignited the eastern sky and showed us to be exactly on course to Shoiba, but still a good few miles away. Thirst was starting to be something which stayed in my consciousness constantly, sparking daydreams of tall glasses of ice cold lemonade, but upon seeing land I knew it wouldn't be long. Unfortunately the current was moving south at a couple of knots, taking us with it, so rather than fight it we decided to land on the south side of the lagoon channel, a mile or so south of the Coast Guard station. But a little after eight we were only about a half mile offshore, but discovered to our dismay that there was a brisk rip current moving away from shore. I tied my gear to my foot, put my head down, and swam freestyle as hard as I could for 30 minutes, thinking any second that I'd bump into shore. When I finally looked up, I couldn't believe my eyes: I'd cleared less than half the distance. I wasn't thinking too clearly at this point, as one might expect (John told me later that at this point he was drifting south and looked back to find me, only to see me running across the top of the waves! Slightly dehydrated!)

Finally, at this frustrating moment, a fishing boat came by with a Saudi fisherman in it. He was perhaps a quarter mile away, running his un-muffled outboard engine wide open, but I let out a holler that would have shattered windows, had there been any within range, so he heard me and circled to pick me up. I shed a few tears of joy and relief, gave my thanks to Allah or whoever it was in charge of that particular sector of the universe, picked up John and rode over to the Coast Guard Station for tea and water.

Since my eyeglasses had been in the boat, I had worn my dive mask (which has my eyeglass prescription built in) and my snorkel for the last 20 hours. Consequently, my lower lip was swollen up like a sausage and my tongue and gums were quite sore. I was stiff all over, and had abrasions on my feet from my fins, and down my arms and neck from my buoyancy compensator. I must have looked quite a sight, as I slowly and awkwardly climbed from the boat and waddled to the coast guard station. One old fellow insisted I drink tea, worrying that plain water would make me vomit. So I drank about a quart of sweet strong tea, which tasted like nectar of the gods at that point. I followed that with a quart of ice water, then slowed down and drank about two more quarts over the next hour. The coast guardians then cooked up a Bedouin feast: lamb on a big plate of rice, eaten sitting cross-legged on the ground. John and I ate a bit, though our thirst far outweighed any hunger.

So I survived the most miserable night of my life – there's not another I can recall even in the same category. And we lost our boat, which presumably floated into the Indian Ocean, which was worth about $2000 at the time. A costly experience in money and suffering. Can Saudi Roddy, the eternal optimist, possibly find any good out of such an event? Of course!

The human body was meant by evolution to travel a rocky road. Climbing through the trees to gather fruit, hunting and running down wild beasts for food, fleeing from larger predators: the life we evolved to live was no picnic. But in the last few hundred years, things have gotten easier and easier, until now we drive the car to the store two blocks away, and take the elevator down one flight. I'm borderline fanatic as far as staying in good physical condition is concerned, but still, you never know how you're are going to react to a challenge until one comes along.

I have always suspected that I was pretty tough: in fact, I think I've been telling everyone that ever since I could talk. But now I have had the opportunity to prove myself to myself, and any hardships in the future will be that much easier to deal with. That macho façade I carry around isn't just bluster: I really can face adversity without complaining. I didn't have any big religious experience: neither God nor Allah nor Jesus nor Muhammad had anything to say to me during my ordeal. But afterward, life was a little more precious, the sky a little bluer, the trees a little greener, my friends a little more appreciated. Minor everyday hassles that everyone bitches about seem unworthy of notice. There's some sort of positive afterglow that slowly fades during the ensuing weeks, but hopefully some small spark will remain.

After my hearing and digesting this astounding tale, I never went into the Red Sea again without a diver's wrist-compass, pressure-proof water canteen and knowledge from the few available, though primitive, maps; and of sun and moon direction, time, temperature and other important navigational parameters. No sea-charts were to be had and this era predated GPS. Also, though I had always exercised religiously and kept in good physical shape, I realized my very survival could depend upon *really* good athletic condition; I upticked workouts big-time. So in addition to five-mile dawn runs daily, dive Fridays excepted, I started regular evening routines, dive Fridays excepted: either another run (up to sixty miles per week total), weight lifting at our tiny hospital gym, or lap-swimming. Al Hada's grounds included a large, well-maintained outdoor pool, circled by a concrete privacy-wall, but strictly segregated with specific hours according to gender, age and marital status. However, it was closed and locked at night, the only time I could swim, free of work.

"Hmm. I can scale that wall."

So I swam my laps secretly, along with occasional other resourceful anonymous folk, in the dark, silently, under a beautiful Arabian desert star-lit sky.

So much for my serene, peaceful initiation into Red Sea life.

The very next Friday brought a new reality onto the scene: *sharks*.
The dive started as pleasant and idyllic as the first. I was beginning to feel at home on twenty-mile-reef, though still hadn't practiced with or carried a gun, but I did drift apart from Rod and John, exploring. A small air-leak developed in my equipment, so I surfaced, and while hanging on to the boat, made the minor repair. I noticed a stringer-line tied to the boat, the stringer dangling several feet below, possibly holding some fish. The line twitched slightly, and I casually mused, "Oh, one of my buddies must be attaching on a new catch."

But then the line suddenly jerked violently, almost capsizing the boat! Instant fright – something terribly wrong! Then a black triangle briefly broke the surface not ten feet from me. (My later comparison: "Just like in an old black-and-white grade B ocean-movie.") I quickly set my mask and ducked undersea just in time to see a large grey shape undulating rapidly away.

Rarely in my life have I panicked, maybe once or twice (never, in a medical situation).

But I panicked at that moment, scrambling back into the boat, eyes wide, breathing hard.

That evening I approached the problem more rationally, as diving was to be my only recreational activity for a year in this strange land.

To myself, "Don't quit. Devise a plan. First, gather all the info possible." I read everything relevant in our little hospital library, interviewed my three dive-buddies, reflected and pondered. Then the plan:
- Constantly alert.
- Become an expert with the gun, keep it always at hand, loaded,

dive-knife strapped to my leg.
- Stay close to the reef, like the small fish do. They know.
- Be aware of the stringer with fish and its attraction for sharks.

The very next Friday my resolve was tested: cruising alone at shallow depth, I spotted a shark about twenty feet ahead, not huge but big enough to cause trouble. He turned, stopped and stared at me with yellow eyes. I thought calmly, "Back against the reef, thumb on the safety (now in the off position), finger on the trigger."

I swear that shark smiled and I could almost hear him thinking, "You silly human! You think I'm interested?" And in a flash he was gone.

Never again did I panic in the Red Sea. But we did encounter sharks, perhaps on half of our dives and I'll recount later some of those adventures.

In all the years following, whenever near the ocean, I think of sharks.

"Oddities"

Over the course of a year, the Red Sea offered up many strange finds.

Once, cruising along near the bottom by a reef, I spied a strange, totally foreign-appearing object: a long, round cylinder-type, maybe fifteen feet in length by two feet thick, partly covered with sand and debris. "It looks like an old water-logged tree trunk," to myself, even a thin vertical-piece sticking straight up for a few feet near the end like an old tree branch. Curious, I reached out and touched the "branch." To my amazement, the "tree" came to life, shook off sand, and twisting, swam slowly off!

Later I described it to John, "What on earth was it?"

John laughed, "That was a nurse shark! Big, ugly, lazy, harmless – they like to sleep on the bottom."

"But why do they call them 'nurse sharks?'"

John only laughed.

(I love telling this story to medical-nurse friends!)

In addition to sharks and the large manta-ray and Portuguese Man-of-War described earlier in Rod's swim-tale, one of the most ferocious underwater beasts is the moray eel; grossly patterned in red-purple-gray-black, some as big as a man's leg. They live in underwater caves and lunge out to strike a fish for dinner, or a human limb.

John first encountered one of these "instruments of the devil." He had just shot a nice-sized redfish and was preparing to store it temporarily on his stringer, when, zoom, a moray sprang out of a camouflaged lair and swallowed the fish whole, in one giant gulp! John, angered at the loss of his nice prize, poked the beast in the belly with his spear – not a traumatic blow but obviously effective, because the Moray regurgitated the whole fish back out! So John recovered his catch, later took it home and cooked it for his own dinner! (Earlier I'd titled this particular vignette, "A Twice-Eaten Fish.")

My first encounter with these "undersea dragons" was a surprise, as unexpectedly he thrust out from a hole in the reef, his head the size of a kid's football, jaw agape – didn't reach my body but almost. I, like John, was angered by this unprovoked assault by such a hideous creature. My first impulse was simply to kill him; I would have loved to shoot him frontally right through that gaping mouth. I envisioned the spear exiting the back of his neck and lodging behind in the reef, he then coiling and writhing about it in death. But then I recalled the warning of Samuel Taylor Coleridge's 1790 epic poem, *The Rime of the Ancient Mariner*; "Woe unto Ye, whosoever wantonly slays God's creatures." So I paused: "Was being vicious, ugly and deadly reason for death?" I mulled the question. Finally mercy prevailed and I simply departed.

(That evening, upon hearing of my undersea ethical-literary-philosophical debate with myself, John absolutely screamed, "Bax, one thing for sure: whenever you argue with yourself, one way or the other, you'll always win!")

89

Sharks! -- My First Kill

It started as a routine dive. Beautiful Friday/weather/water/fish/coral! At the reef, I had wandered away from buddies in this silent undersea splendor, but then a minor problem with my spear-gun. So I climbed back into the boat, removed and hung the vest-plus-attached air tank onto a hook at the outer gunwale, it now dangling in the water. Off with mask-snorkel, flippers remaining on.

Now to unload the gun and make repairs.

After a few minutes, task completed, I reach for the vest-tank, but gone! It had worked loose from the hook in the gentle boat-rocking and floated away, buoyed by the air tank and caught in the strong currents tailing around the reef! It was rapidly disappearing over the horizon – my five-hundred-dollar American dive vest! Startled; then quick to retrieval; no time to load a spear; quickly into mask-snorkel and over the side.

Then, surface-swimming alone in the open ocean, no bottom in sight, fast with the strong current, legs only, unarmed, holding my gun but uselessly unloaded, the spear trailing fifteen feet behind on its tether-line.

I think, "Oh, boy. All I need now is a shark!"

And if by magic – or *fate* – suddenly there appears one, about twenty feet below me! He wasn't big, smaller than me, but big enough to cause trouble, obviously interested but not threatening. He would occasionally roll up a bit on his side and stare at me with yellow eyes, then dart out away but always come back.

Finally, finally, I reach my vest-with-air tank, loop an arm through it, "pull a one-eighty," now trudging back slowly against the fast current. Mr. Shark dutifully turns also, clearly intrigued but not excited or attacking. Finally – finally! I reach the reef, now my back to it, quickly load the gun with both bands for maximum power. I notice a stringer with bleeding fish dangling in the water from our nearby boat. "Good! Now he'll get interested in that shark-treat and forget about me."

Sure enough, he circles the stringer, faster, becoming excited by the blood, but instead of charging the stringer, he threatens me! Circling, then at me but turning away, faster, repeating, but lastly straight at me, mouth agape!

I shot him in the chest at point-blank range.

He spun violently away, the spear-point lodged deeply, snapping the tether-line to my gun. My buddy Mark, who had now approached and was hovering near the surface, shot him again and the shark fell dead to the ocean floor.

I breathed a sigh of relief, but for me no celebration or chest-beating. I had entered his ocean-world where he has ruled, archeologists tell us, for millions of years.

But my survival instincts prevailed.

So I killed my first shark while surface-swimming, one arm through the vest-with-tank, firing with one hand from the hip, Rambo-style.

Thenceforth whenever in the sea, sharks become at once, "the first thing I look for and the last thing I want to see."

"Big Ones"

Occasionally John would mumble under his breath, totally out of context with anything currently being discussed, "Someday the big one [i.e., shark] will come in."

On September 16, 1983, mid-morning at five-mile reef, John, Mark and I at about thirty-feet depth, it happened.

Only it wasn't the big one – it was two big ones! I don't know for sure their size, not giant, but each bigger than me (six-feet three-inches tall, one-hundred eighty-five pounds). Strangely, as identified by markings, they were two different breeds: one a white-tipped "oceanic" shark, the other a ferocious mako, which appeared first. Initially I didn't see him. John did, later describing with laughter my sudden terrified expression as I glanced over my shoulder, and, "Oh, S -- !" (It is not my style to use obscenities; they are simply some feeble, desperate tools of the ignorant, hoping to shock you. But in this situation, one obscenity in particular seemed not only permissible, but demanded. I mouthed it around my snorkel.) As written in my dive-log that evening, "He circled me three times," obviously interested, but thankfully not threatening or attacking, so I refrained from shooting. (My dive-routine for protection against sharp coral included wearing long sleeves, blue-jeans and gloves in addition to dive-equipment; later I wondered if I appeared too "wrapped" for his appetite.)

He departed in a flash.

"Whew!"

But next came the big "oceanic"!
After spotting him, I glanced over and saw Mark crouched behind a coral tower, staring, eyes almost bigger than his goggles! John was near, close to his stringer of fish which happened to be tied to his wrist. In a flash the big one raced by, grabbed the entire stringer in his powerful jaws, pulling John along at speed by his wrist! The water flew by John's face so fast the flutter-valve on his mask jammed, making breathing difficult. But somehow, in spite of all this, he got off a remarkable shot with one hand, hitting the shark just behind the head! The beast swallowed the many fish on the stringer and then spit it out, now a tangled-mangled piece of metal. Putting on a further burst of speed, the shark snapped the tether-line attaching

spear-head to gun without even slowing, now freeing John from tow. This "big one" was last seen heading to the open ocean, blood streaming from the spear tip impaled in his side.

His last meal would be a tasty one.

We three climbed back into the boat, the only time ever quitting with air still in our tanks, the only time ever I glimpsed a hint of fear in John's steel-grey eyes.

Poseidon, the Greek Sea-God

Our Red Sea, in contrast to such waters as the North Sea (about the UK and continental Europe) or the South China Sea, does not have a reputation of severe storms. Indeed, as we traversed between shore and our favorite reefs aboard dive-boat "Barracuda", often hardly a ripple patterned the surface. Any sailboat might have been forever becalmed. Even past land-sight, the Red Sea was often as a pond. No Storms.

Except once.

Occasionally our hospital had official foreign visitors: doctors, technical advisors, business types, etc. (All visitors must be "official" and carefully screened. No tourists are allowed into the country. Visas are required before boarding any in-bound plane. Also, maybe there were some, but I never saw a female visitor.) Sometimes I would hear that said visitor was a diver. Then I would ask John, "I think he's a 'scuba' – shouldn't we invite him along next trip?" John, not exactly knowing how to spell the word *humility*, would reply, "If he's really good, he'll find us." So we rarely had a dive-guest, though we did on this particular day.

On May 20, late AM., I cruised around the corner of the reef alone, as was our practice, at about thirty-feet depth, heading back to the boat. My air was low and I towed a stringer of fish. Time to consider home. Approaching *Barracuda* from below, I was mystified to see the anchor-line shaking violently; alternating totally lax, sagging, coiling on the bottom, then suddenly tight and straight-vertical. Looking up, I saw the boat rising and falling precipitously – huge waves! Quickly up and into it, with difficulty, my whole world now taking on a new dimension. The others, John, Rod and visitor, soon followed; we weighed anchor and anxiously started back toward land.

My sea-experience limited, I had never encountered anything even approaching this storm – a full gale, tremendous wind and waves, but strangely blue skies above. Though no rain, the air seemed almost as solid water, fierce wind blowing wave-tops horizontally, we all wearing our dive masks even now above surface. The waves were huge, each topped with a giant foaming roll of surf. The only way we could navigate toward shore was to aim straight into each roller, the bow now pointing

94

up to the sky, but then to bear off to the right as we then rode downhill into the next massive swell.* John at the wheel; the wind so extreme and loud that the only way I could communicate with him was to place my mouth exactly at his ear and then scream as loudly as possible. (I recalled Joseph Conrad's epic storm-tale, *Typhoon*, wherein Captain MacWhirr could only communicate with his first-mate in this self-same manner.)**

I knew the worry was hitting one of these massive breakers at the wrong angle – the wave would then roll us, broach, and *Barracuda* would go down stern-first, weighted by the motor. But being a swimmer and at home in the warm waters of the Red Sea, I knew my chance of making shore, visible several miles distant, was good, even through this raging storm, particularly wearing my dive equipment. I was confident of John and Rod, too, though unsure about the visitor.

Finally, finally we limped ashore, the motor missing badly from water intake, miles south of our usual inlet. I kissed our trusty *Barracuda* on the nose as we tied her to a tree; here she could sleep 'til our next foray. Hopefully the Sea-God Poseidon won't be so angry then!

We caught a ride with some locals back to our SUV and, exhausted, ate up those miles back to Taif and the hospital, my desert-home.

But for me, this storm-drama wasn't yet over. After a night of dreamless, deep sleep, I awaken, totally startled and alert in the pre-dawn darkness and at once euphoric:

"I'm a livin' man!"

* In all the years to follow, I am reminded of these waves whenever in a sports-arena or multi-level auditorium – such was their immensity.

** Later I laughed at myself, bothering to recall classic literature at a time of personal danger!

This mantra keeps reverberating in my mind. Jumping out of bed, into running clothes (long pants and sleeves – no immodest dress in Saudi), through the door, onto the well-lit but now empty freeway, the start of my daily five-mile loop, I am pathologically happy after yesterday's almost-tragedy: "I'm a livin' man!" Bounding by a family of wild dogs in the desert (no house pets permitted), the pups playing in the sand, the parents sitting on their haunches, staring at me with eyes glowing like coals in the dark.

"Hi, dogs! Top o' the mornin' to ya!" I run backward! I skip!
A wild camel, munching early breakfast on desert shrubs, regards me with baleful brown eyes. "Good morning, Mister Camel! You think I'm crazy? Well, I am! I'm a livin' man!"

I pass a water-truck, tending trees along, the workers staring, shaking heads; I almost hear their thoughts, "What goof is that, running along the freeway at dawn?" (Occasionally, in my daybreak running, a local, unused to seeing us weird types, would burst out of his house and stare behind me; for surely if a man is running down the street, someone, or some thing, must be chasing him!)

Finally past the four-mile mark, my cranked-up metabolism has burned away all those euphoria-producing endorphins, and I return to emotional near-normality, ready to begin the climb up that final half-mile grade, aptly named "nausea hill." I had started forty-minutes earlier in total darkness, but now, near the equator, bright sun prevails ("The dawn comes up like thunder," wrote Rudyard Kipling.) The northeast on-shore wind brings warm moist air over from the Red Sea, which hits our higher elevation, cools, forms a cloud and is brightened by the emerging sun; the result is a beautiful pink-purple fog rolling up onto the freeway each morning – a welcome distraction for this upper altitude, panting runner. Now past the modest palace of Harvard-educated Saudi Oil Minister Sheikh Ahmed Yamani,* then – finish. Recovery, thence to our small apartment. A standard breakfast of blended raw eggs (complete with shells), yogurt, wheat germ and fruit; clean-up; then into scrub-clothes together with wool sweater ("You silly runners are forever cold!"); and now I'm ready for another day of –

"Life in the hospital."

*Legend has it that decades earlier, Sheik Yamani had visited Paris, France. From his hotel balcony, he gazed down upon the huge city with its bustling, congested motor-traffic and mused, "Look at all those vehicles burning our oil." He then reflected upon his own Saudi citizens, mostly either Bedouin nomads wandering the desert with their goats and camels, or poor village shop-keepers trying to eke out survival with the barest of infrastructure, education and health care.

He pondered this disparity awhile.

Then the Sheik stated, "I think I'll triple the price of oil."

And the world has never been the same since.

Home

Toward the end of 1983, my year in Saudi Arabia is closing. John drives me to Jedda's international airport.

"Bax, will you dive again?"

My eyes moisten. I don't answer.

("It will only make you miss the Red Sea and your buddies.

You'll never be this good a diver again.

Most dive-places don't even permit spear-guns, let alone these big harpoons.") *

A short hop over the Red Sea; detained transiently by Egyptian Police for uttering an obscenity about a certain regional political figure. (Should have known better – "Everywhere ain't the USA.")

Overnight with old friends in Cairo.

Then the joyous, joyous, joyous flight out of the Middle East, the alcohol flowing freely, my boots stuffed with hundred-dollar bills, over the pyramids, over the Mediterranean, over the Alps, (invited to the flight-deck for the view, this before the Age of Terrorism), we descend into the Christmas ambiance of Merrie London. I attend a performance of the Royal Ballet. Tears flow down my cheeks (to the surprise of the Brits about me – it wasn't *that* good a performance – but they hadn't just "yeared" in the Muslim desert.)

*I never dove again. Only later, while reflecting back upon my life-altering year in Saudi Arabia, did I associate that memorable one-word conclusion to Edgar Allan Poe's famous poem, *The Raven*:

"Nevermore."

Then home, standing alone in my small apartment, Birmingham, unoccupied for exactly one year.

"He's crazy," my friends would say. "Give him time. He'll re-adjust."

But you're used to different colors, rhythms, sounds, values, tones – different hues, smells, shapes, moves, feels –

I suppose the green hills of Birmingham will be the closest thing to "home" that I will ever know. But even now, years later, in running these soft, silent hills alone at daybreak, the wheels of my memory often roll back to other dawns a third of the world to the east, and I relive once again those wild undersea adventures with John, Rod and Mark, in the savage virgin splendor of the Red Sea reefs south of Jedda, "almost any Friday, 1983."

-- Written 1992

The Desert

The cold winds and hot sands
   extract a toll
         from each who tread these desert paths.
Blown away are the games,
   the ritual, the façade --
And though the body is clothed,
   the soul stands naked and visible.
For there is no gray here,
   only black and white,
      hate and love,
         death and life.
So let the passer-by be forewarned:
   he will experience the beauty,
      but he will pay the price.
A different reality is confronted.
He can never see the world
   through the same eyes again,
And his life is changed forever.

(Saudi Arabia, 1983)

ILLUSTRATIONS

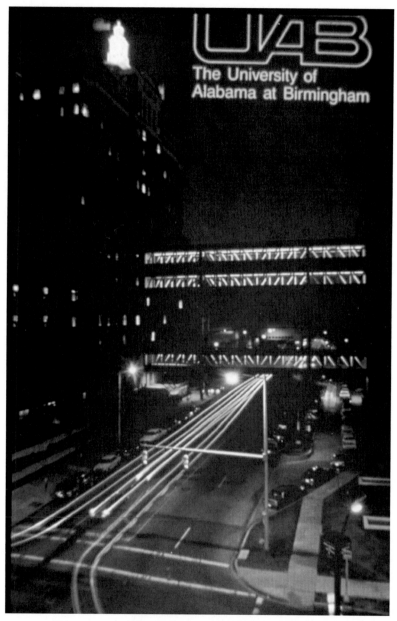

University Hospital, Birmingham, Alabama; my home for most of those thirty-five years a medical doctor.

Coronary artery by-pass grafting, starting in the late1960s, has literally saved the lives and improved symptoms of millions wordwide. (Notice surgical vein-harvesting from the leg, upper-left in this photo. That vein-segment will then be sewed in place to provide bypass blood-flow around a blockage.) Newer techniques now are less traumatic for certain cases, and balloon angioplasty permits non-surgical blockage correction in selected patients.

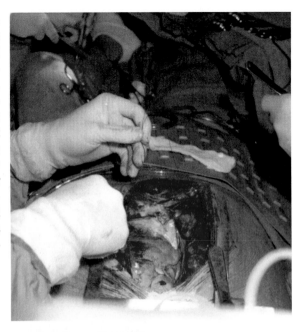

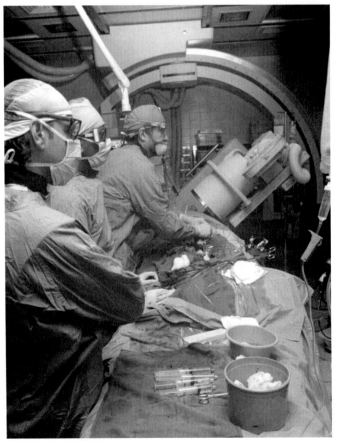

Percutaneous transluminal coronary angioplasty (PTCA) involves snaking balloon-catheters and other devices up to the heart from the femoral (groin) blood vessels under x-ray guidance. We balloon-types were jokingly referred to as "plumbers" because of our roto-rooter mentality, in contrast to "electricians" -- cardiologists specializing in rhythm-distubance treatment with medications, pacemakers and other devices and treatments.

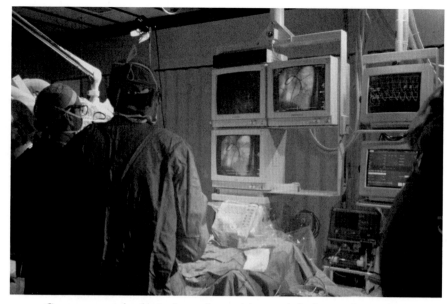

Coronary angioplasty is performed in semi-darkness for optimal x-ray visualization on the black-and white monitors. The screens to the right display real-time physiologic data, also requiring continuous attention.

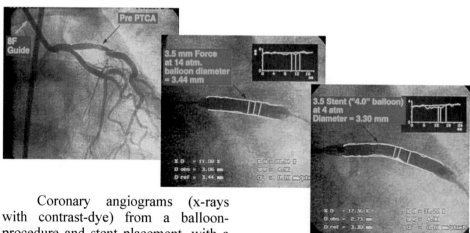

Coronary angiograms (x-rays with contrast-dye) from a balloon-procedure and stent placement, with a software program displaying the vessel diameter. Panel A shows thenarrowing before treatment; then the initial balloon inflation, B, squeezing the blockage-material (cholesterol-plaque) back into the vessel wall; C displays the stent deployment to prop the artery open during healing; and finally D, our end result. (The stent itself is barely visible.)

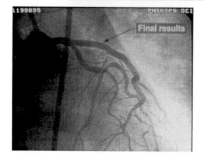

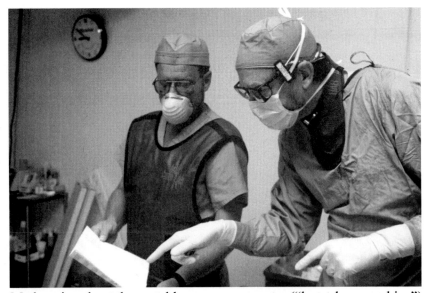

My learning about the portable pump-oxygenator ("heart-lung machine") from a perfusionist (expert operator, in green), both courtesy of our Surgery Department, during a high-risk angioplasty procedure. Mechanical circulatory-support systems interested me, a holdover from earlier years as an engineer. We were one of few angioplasty institutions worldwide utilizing that particular technology.

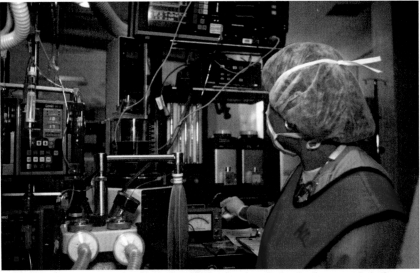

Routine coronary angioplasty is relatively simple in design, straightforward and uncomplicated, utilizing mild sedation and local anesthesia only. However, more-risky procedures may involve multiple high-technology devices with skilled teams of personnel-operators, general anesthesia and mechanical circulatory-assistance. Research protocols may be followed also, adding another layer of complexity.

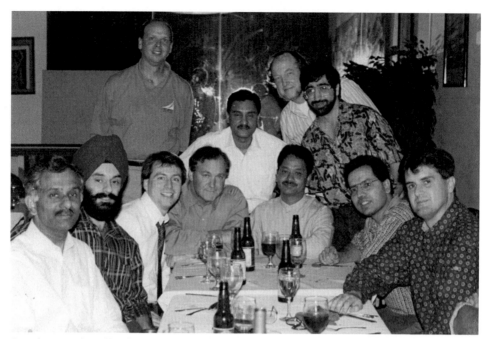

Our internationally-flavored UAB Interventional (i.e. "balloon angioplasty") Cardiologists, both staff-attendings and fellows-in-training, 1990s. Our Director was Gary Roubin, MD PhD (seated, blue), with Larry Dean, MD (standing, red) second in command. (That's me behind, bending.)

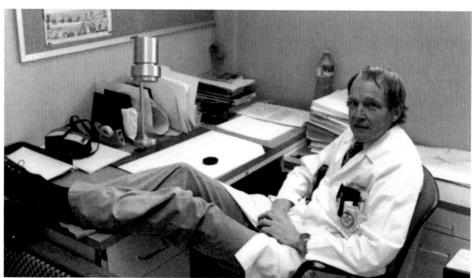

My modest office in Al Hada Hospital, City of Taif, Kingdom of Saudi Arabia, 1983. It was a good, medium-sized teaching hospital serving the general populace. The official language was English, with translators everywhere, mostly Lebanese, speaking fluent Arabic, English and French.

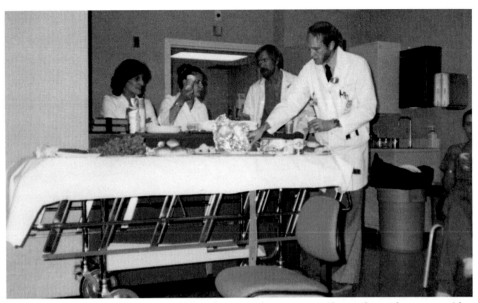

"No patient? No problem! We'll just have an impromptu 'brunch on the gurney' by a few of our multi-national Saudi cardiology team." Note the women with hair uncovered, permissible only in certain settings. (That's me, choosing.) No alcoholic beverages available anywhere in The Kingdom. However, a few of us resourceful types made wine for off-call evening enjoyment, "– a bit cloudy, but aged a full two weeks."

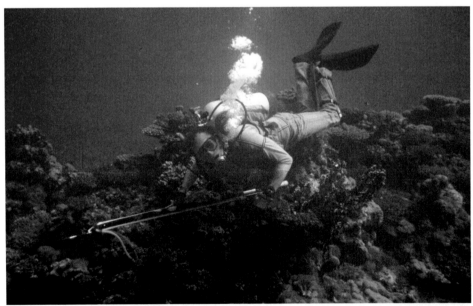

Scuba-diving the Red Sea, most Fridays the entirety of 1983; this plus work-outs my only regular activities besides doctoring. Note the size of the gun, more harpoon than spear-gun. Dive-buddy John Cooney bought them on a recent trip to Australia, near the Great Barrier Reef.

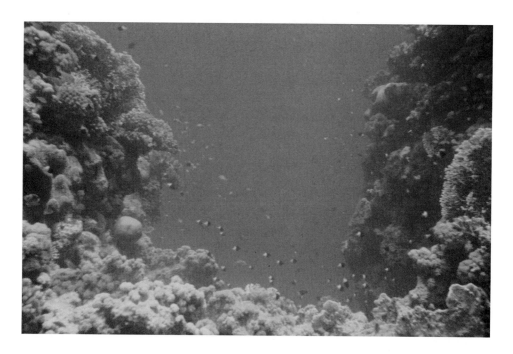

My underwater camera, even with "color film," nevertheless failed (upper panel) to reproduce the spectacular hues of Red Sea coral visible while diving. Lower panel reveals the same image after high-tech color enhancement, artistically recreated according to my memory.

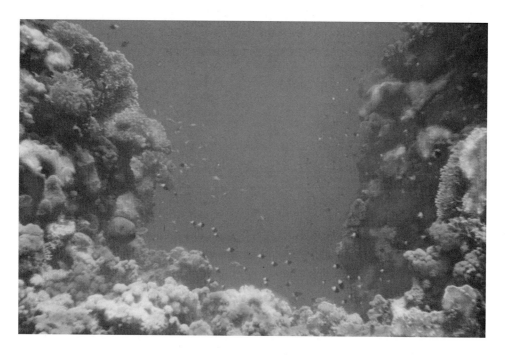

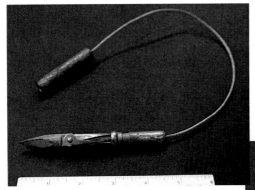

These two images with inch-scales demonstrate the break-away point and then fold-back barbs on the spears for our scuba guns. Once lodged in a fish – or other underwater-thing – the barbs opened and it stayed, with a tether-line back to the diver for retrieval of his prize.

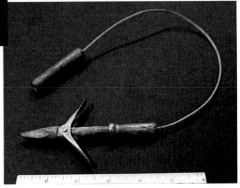

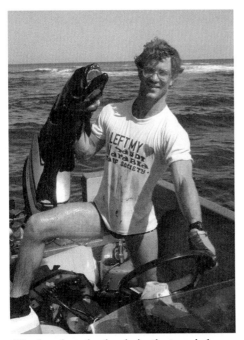

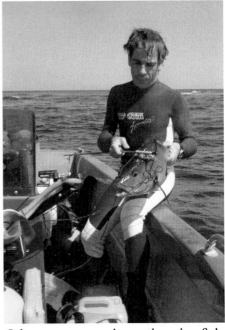

"Rod, what-the-heck is that weird creature you shot?" I forget his answer, but in the course of diving a "year of Fridays", we encountered many a weird creature in the Red Sea. (See text.)

John removes a nice eating-size fish from his spear-tip. No wonder sharks found him interesting, so colorful! (I was drab in comparison, but on occasion they hassled me also.)

108

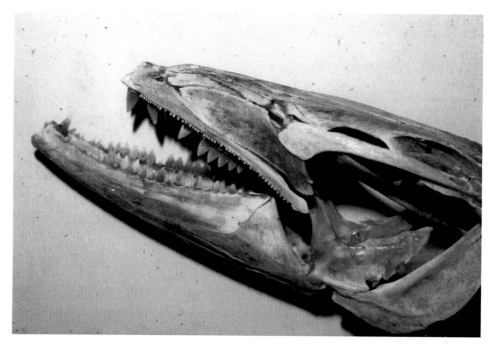

This scary photo tells a funny story: John had never taken formal dive-training, was self-taught. Some weeks before my arrival into Saudi, he had shot a large bar-racuda. In the city of Jedda, surprisingly, there existed a combination of dive-shop, certification-center and sea-life taxidermy, mainly to serve divers north of town (our exclusive domain was south). John took this fish-head in to be processed into a display-memento, but first he asked the shop-manager if he could be certified, since he was now an experienced diver. "Sorry, you'll first have to take a qualifica-tion course."

"Oh well, okay, I understand. But another question: here's the head of a barracuda I shot. Can you process it into a display-skull for me?" (This photographed result is the size of a "kid's football" – it measured nine inches tall before collapsing into a pile of dust years later.)

The store-owner stared at the head, then went to his desk and started writing.

"What are you doing?" asked John.

"Filling out your dive-certification. Anyone who could kill a barracuda that big is a qualified diver!"

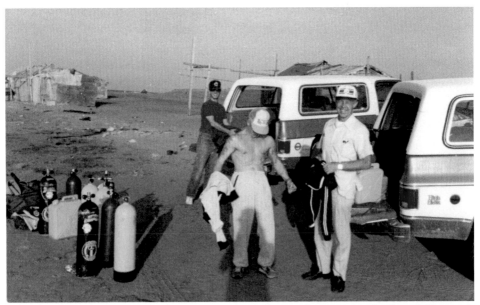

Anticipating our upcoming Red Sea scuba-dive, John gets excited and "hams it up" on the beach.

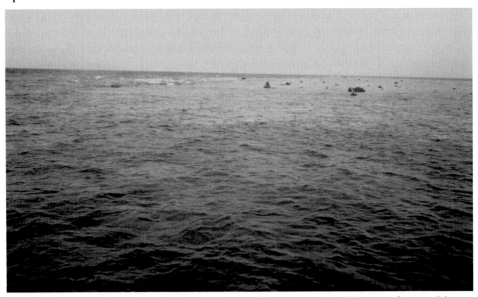

This dreary, uninteresting-looking picture of the empty Red Sea surface, with occasional coral outcroppings in this particular location, nevertheless depicts the beginning of an amazing saga. This is what John and Rod saw, in every direction, after the two emerged following a dive shortly before my arrival in Saudi, realized that their dive-boat was gone, had drifted away, and that they were bobbing up and down alone in the open ocean ten miles from shore, with no chance of rescue! (See text for their spellbinding story. "I – can't imagine – how it must have felt.")

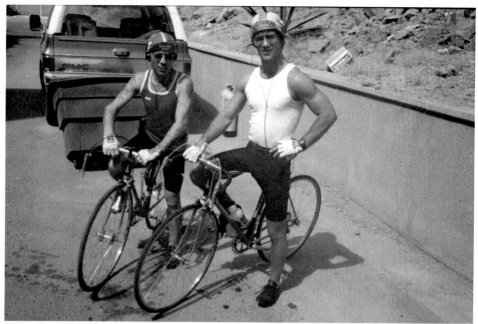

Being in top physical condition literally saved the lives of these two divers: John Cooney, RN (red) and Rodney Groomes, MD (white). See text.

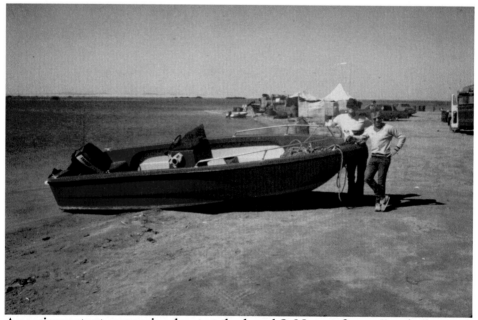

An unimportant-appearing boat at the beach? Not so for us "scuba" types! This, our beloved dive-boat *Barracuda*, saved us during that terrible sea-storm (see text).

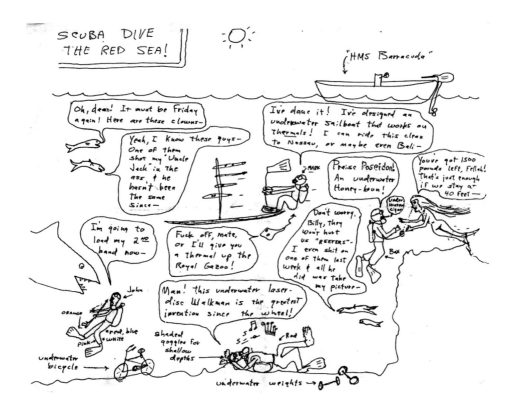

I drew this spoof of us four divers and some of our favorite themes in Saudi Arabia, 1983. (Please accept my apologies for the obscenities – the only ones in this entire book, and for the tiny print, necessary for publication.) "Jack" refers to amberjack, a spirited and tasty game-fish at our reefs: they could grow large and at times after being shot could tow rapidly one – or even two! – divers awhile by the tether-lines attached to our spear-tips. John's "two bands" means loading his gun for maximum power, needed for large fish and sharks. (Poseidon is the mythical Greek sea-God. I later made this one-word substitution from another diety to avoid offending local folk.) Mark was a sailboat enthusiast, Rod liked music and physical work-outs, and John dressed in color and seemed forever tangling with sharks.

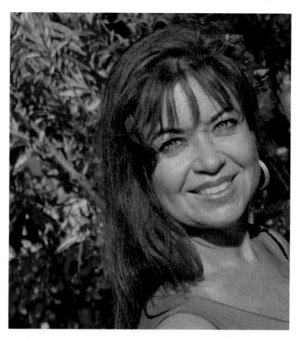

Patricia Boswell RN tended the severely ill in UAB Hospital's Coronary Care Unit while I doctored in Taif, Saudi Arabia, all of 1983. ("Doesn't she look Cuban?" [See text.])

Later we would wed.

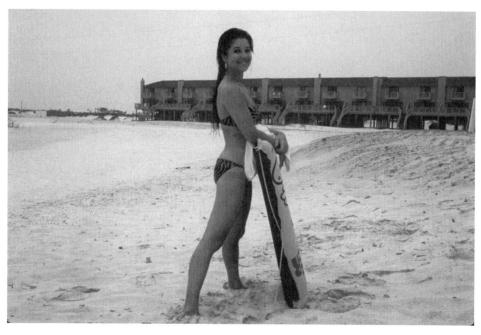

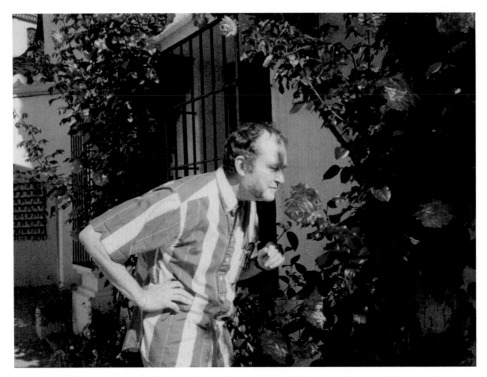

Nineteen-ninety-seven, almost sixty-five years old, complex multi-vessel coronary angioplasty with stents in severely ill patients day/night while the technology raced ahead at 100 MPH: no work for old men. (A forty-year-old quarterback?) Time to stop, quit, exhale, retire, smell the roses, reflect back on all that hospital drama, then write a much-needed book.

BOOK TWO

FICTION

"That Two-Eyed Girl's Weather Report"

Screenplay

(Scene – Interior of a workout gymnasium. Contemporary. Soft background music. A young man in workout clothes, exercising, is the narrator -- a voiceover -- with the action he describes depicted simultaneously and silently on the screen.)

Narrator: "So there I was, pedaling a stationary bicycle, reading an abbreviated Shakespeare's play "Twelfth Night" in e-book format so I could enlarge the font to prevent squinting while bouncing on the bike.

I hardly noticed another rider climbing onto the next bike. But then I did a double-take, looking again, staring, thinking, 'Wow, check that out!' I didn't have to search for words – they just tumbled into my brain like cubes into a glass from an ice maker: 'Statuesque, busty, curvy, young, maybe twenties, moderately tall and muscular, a great bod, maybe an athlete or dancer or both, tight tee-shirt and thankfully no tattoos or wedding ring. But, rather unkempt long red hair tied in back, a pretty face though poor make-up, ragged workout cut-offs and what looks like dancers' practice slippers, no socks. Also, something about her intensity of gaze further intrigued me, even there in the boring ambiance of early-evening workouts.'"

He: "Haven't seen you around here before. You a new member of the club?"

Narrator: "She hardly glanced at me, paused, then in a voice I found rather husky – and sexy, like the rest of her. "

She: "Trying it out before joining."

He: "It's a funny old club, dates back over a century. But equipment, pool and track are good, locker rooms clean. And notice all the historic photos on the wall with old newspaper clippings."

Narrator: "I climbed off and tried to keep our little dialog going."

He: "If I can help you with any of these work-out machines, let me know. Some of them are kind of cantankerous. I'll be over there, arm weights."

She: "Thanks."

Narrator: "Later, after showered and dressed, I headed out. But through the front glass doors I could see a downpour. She stood just inside, obviously dismayed. Now I had hopes."

"Oh, heavens! Are you walking?"

"Yes."

"I have a car, but don't even want to run to the parking lot in this rain.

116

I have an idea – you may have seen our little club-bar in the back. How about we go there, I buy you a drink. This will let up soon and then I'll drive you home."

(She looks him up and down carefully, then,) "Okay."

Narrator: "We perched on bar stools, she a martini, I iced tea. I silently thanked fate for this encounter."

(He, extending his hand,) "I'm Royal Grace. Call me Roy."

"Nice to meet you. Aida Saint Cyr."

(They shake hands.)

"Aida, like in the opera?"

"Just like it."

"A wow-name! Are you Egyptian too? As I recall, she was a slave-girl who gets sealed up in a cave with her boyfriend at the end. Not exactly a happy way to conclude a relationship."

"Not Egyptian and never had a chance to see opera."

"Seems I've heard your name somewhere."

"Maybe out front of the Paradise Bar on Bourbon Street. I dance there."

Narrator: "Oh, this is interesting! Thanks, fate."

"Is that a stage name?"

"It started out that way, but then I changed it to official. My birth name was April May."

"You do have interesting names!"

"My mother must have had a sense of humor."

"Dancer at a bar – that sounds like exciting work."

"It has its ups and downs, if you know what I mean. The money with tips has been good. But I just quit."

"What happened?"

"It's a long story."

"That's okay; you don't have to explain. My life's a bit less exciting. I'm a second year medical student over at the university. Study-study. I'm not much fun these days. Kind of a nerd."

"Oh, you're going to become a doctor?"

"Hopefully."

"That's wonderful. Your life will lead somewhere. Mine doesn't look too promising. (Pause) I think the rain has stopped. Thanks for offering to drive me home."

(They now in his car, a residential neighborhood.)

"There it is, third house on the left. Oh, oh, bad news – that's my suitcase on the porch. Looks like I don't live here anymore."

"What's going on?"

"I didn't want to get into all this, it's kind of personal, but here goes: that's the boss's house. He gives me a room as benefit with my job, but now says I have to – how should I say – be intimate with him, to keep the job plus room. So I quit. Looks like he's throwing me out today. You can let me off here. I'll get my stuff and walk over to the YWCA. They'll give me a room temporarily and I'll be safe there."

"Here, I can help and then drive you to the 'Y'."

(She exits the car and climbs to the porch while he parks. As she picks up her suitcase, the boss emerges through the front door, speaking angrily,) "You bitch! I'm giving you one last chance to keep your job and room, even a raise, but on my terms!" (He grabs her wrist roughly.)

"No! I'm leaving."

(Roy approaches quickly, defiantly.) "Don't you touch her!"

"Who the hell are you? Back off!" (Continues to hold her wrist.)

"Let her go! I'm warning you – I have a black belt in Tai Kwan Do."

(Laughing,) "Oh the rescuing knight in armor, eh? Right out of the movies! I have a belt, too, with something in it." (Reaches behind himself and pulls a handgun, keeps it pointed upward,) Now you two clear out before I get angry."

(They, wide-eyed, quickly retreat, enter his car, depart.)

(He, grimacing,) "Wow! Ragged character! Glad you're leaving."

"Oh, I'm sorry you got mixed up in all this, but if you could drop me off at the 'Y,' I'd 'appreciate it."

"Sure, although it's past dinner time. Why not stop off at my place first. It's close-by and I've got some good left-over pizza."

(She stares at him, uncertain, cautious, then,) "Alright."

(They enter his small apartment, she with suitcase.)

"Welcome. Bathroom down the hall, left."

"Oh, look at all your books! You must be smart."

"I like to read, but med-school is pretty demanding – not much otherwise these days."

"I always wanted to read books, but Mother took me out of school on my sixteenth birthday and put me to work. Been working ever since. No time for other stuff."

(New scene, later, they relaxing in his living room after supper.)

118

Aida: "Good pizza and beer. You've been kind to me. Thank you."

"No problem. Why don't you just rest here a moment? I have to make some phone calls about school for a few minutes and then I'll drive you." (Exits to bedroom.)

(Later, he returns; she is now asleep, semi-reclining to the side against pillows.)

Narrator, speaking softly to himself: "Be careful, Roy. She's a handful and complicated. Remember, you don't really know her. Sometimes bad people appear okay at first."

(He gently removes her shoes and lifts her feet onto the couch, pulls away one of the pillows so she reclines more evenly, she moaning slightly but not awakening. He covers her with a thin blanket and turns off the light.)

(Next morning, bright sunshine through windows. She awakens abruptly, wide-eyed, stares about, rubs her eyes, sees a large cardboard sign propped up on a chair, large letters: "Good morning! Hope you slept well. Make yourself at home. Food in fridge and pantry, towels in bath closet, help yourself to any books. I'll be home after eight PM. If you go out, please leave keys under mat. Hope you'll stay at least another night. I'll even provide sheets!

-- Roy"

(New scene. That evening. He enters his apartment, tired, in medical scrub-clothing.

She greets him, colorfully dressed with an apron, animated and sparkling.)

"Welcome home! Hope you had a nice day."

"Pretty much wiped out. Pathology. It is engrossing, though. Very basic. The anatomy, physiology and biochemistry of disease. Autopsies. Interesting, but work. All day. Finally finished. Do you know how to make a martini?"

"Do I? You're looking at the world's greatest – in my limited opinion, anyway. I was a bartender in Keokuk, Iowa for awhile. Served those Mississippi River boatmen, a tough bunch but nice to me. I'll bet you'd like to try one of my inventions: anchovy instead of olive."

(Later, both relaxing in the living room, Roy, with martini,) "And how was your day?

"Oh heavens, best day I can recall! Slept in, worked out, cleaned house – didn't disturb anything – washed my hair, read books all afternoon. I made lasagna for our dinner. I figured if you like pizza, you'd like lasagna."

"Good grief, you're amazing!"

(Next AM, early. Roy awakens in bed, arises slowly, into a bathrobe, stumbles to the living room. She and her belongings are gone, bedding folded. He sees a hand-written note on the table: "Dear Roy, Thank you for your kindness to me when I was pretty much floundering.

I'm leaving town.

I just know you'll become a good doctor and help people in need.

God bless you, Aida."

(He sighs deeply, sits on the sofa, eyes closed, chin on chest, hand to forehead,) "Damn. Damn."

(New scene, He stands in front of Aida's boss's house, rings the bell. "Boss" appears, recognizes Roy, puts his hands up, grimaces,) "Hey, before you say anything, I'm sorry for the way I treated you both the other day. Running a bar on Bourbon Street is pretty ragged. You interact with bad characters on a regular basis and sometimes it rubs off on me, unfortunately. I hope you guys forgive me.

Please, come in."

(They enter. The boss closes his door.)

"Let me guess: she left."

"Yes. This morning. I'm trying to find where she went, wanted to ask you if she ever mentioned family. Also, thanks for your apology. Life gets harsh sometimes."

"I remember once she mentioned she had no family, and on her employment application, under 'emergency contact,' she put 'none.'"

"Looks like I'm at a dead end."

"Wish I could help you but I can't. If you do see her, tell her I'm sorry and if she ever wants her old job back, she can have it with no strings attached, plus a raise.

I have to tell you, I've been in this business for twenty years and I've learned the ropes. These bar-dancers are a diverse and interesting bunch. The good ones do well with tips, but all drift on after awhile. Some are overt prostitutes, and at the other end, some are married family women with kids. Some are even college students working their way. I once had a writer who wanted to 'experience life.' And a few lesbians, believe it or not, and I actually tried out a transgender once, but he-she got booed off the stage! I never know why, but many dancers seem to choose boyfriends who knock them around, are cruel. Also, the druggies and drinkers – I kick them out fast. And some are illegal aliens, living under cover. But Aida was different. She seemed to have more to her than most, thought about stuff, asked questions, which most people don't. I liked her."

(Two weeks later. Roy returns home at night, alone in his car, steady cold rain. As he turns into the driveway, he sees something on his front step, can't make it out in darkness and rain. As he approaches, realizes it's a person, sitting hunched beneath a large umbrella against the rain.

She looks up, he recognizes her,) "Aida! Good grief! Come in!" (He helps her stand; they enter, she with suitcase,) "You're back! So glad to see you! Missed you." (He embraces her warmly, then studies her closely. She is wet-streaked in rain, shivering, disheveled.) "What happened? You look terrible!"

"I'd rather not talk about it. I went to Las Vegas. It didn't work out."

"It's okay. No problem. What do you want first, a drink, a bath, or dinner?"

"If you're offering, I'll take all three, in that order."

"You've got it! We have nice beef stew for dinner, with good red wine to celebrate your coming home. Missed you – missed you."

"I'm not sure where my home is, but have to admit this place feels good.)

(Later, after dinner, still at the table)
Roy: "Some school friends are having a little party tomorrow evening, celebrating Pathology finals. If you want to, we can go. You'll like them."

"I don't have any nice clothes. "

"Oh, you'll be okay – they're all pretty laid back."

(New scene, festive, a simply-furnished small apartment, evening. Twenty or so students and guests, a diverse young group, attractive, casually dressed, sport shirts, colorful dresses, some blue jeans; drinking variously;

121

munching snacks and finger food; moderately noisy; a happy, convivial party.

One girl in the group, whispering to another,) "Look, Roy came with a new date. I wonder what Sandra thinks about that!"

"Oh, they broke up. He overheard her talking on her cell-phone, saying she hoped their relationship worked out because she wanted to be a doctor's wife. He got really angry at that, said, 'You're an attractive girl, I'm sure you'll find some chump of a medical student or house-officer who doesn't know he's being used.'"

(Aida converses with a small group of guests – they obviously curious about her. She's "different.")

Guest: "So your mom was gone a lot?"

"Sure was. I still don't know what she was doing. We had hardly anything, no money, no other family. Then she took me out of school when I turned sixteen, had my tubes tied and put me to work – been working since. I left home shortly after that. No more school."

"Had your tubes tied? Prevent pregnancy?"

"Yes. Afraid I was a pretty wild teenager."

"And now you've been a stripper at a bar on Bourbon St. That must be a different life."

"Ha, ha, we prefer the term 'exotic dancer'. It is interesting for awhile. I like those college boys and the military guys as customers – they get all excited at a female body, 'whoop!' and stomp their feet. And the older types are fun, too, make 'em smile and feel young again. The bad parts are those weird-o's who stumble into the bar at two AM, think they can do anything to a dancer. That's why I pack heat."

"Pack heat?"

"That means carry a loaded handgun in my purse. It's small, thirty-two caliber, only five rounds, actually a single-action Colt revolver. Would you like to see it? The safety is on."

"Oh, no!"

"I took a course in self defense awhile back, go to the firing range every few months. If you're going to be armed, you'd better know how. I've not fired it in defense, but have had to brandish it – I think that's the right word – take it out, pointed at the ceiling. You never want to point a gun at someone unless you plan to kill him. Usually showing it alone will send a bad guy heading out quick. But I just quit that job as dancer. Had some issues with the boss."

"And now you live with Roy Grace?"

"We must be careful with word choice. I'm a temporary house guest.

I sleep on the couch. Have been enjoying his books 'til I make my next move. They are wonderful! History, literature, even poetry – have you ever heard of e.e. cummings, the poet?"

"An exotic dancer who reads e.e. cummings?"

"Wait, I do read him, but sure I can't understand him! I'll need some help with that. For starters, he never uses capitol letters, even in his name."

(As she was discoursing, other guests, mixed, though mostly women, wide-eyed, had formed a loose circle about her. She, suddenly aware of this,) "Excuse me." (Breaks away, finds Roy,) "Maybe we can leave soon."

"Sure. Anything wrong?"

"Don't know, but it's best."

"Okay."

(New scene, they in his car, headed home. She, distraught, hand to her forehead,) "Oh, good move, Aida." (Then looking at him,) "You're the first guy in my life with something to him who has been nice to me, and I reward you by embarrassing you in front of your friends. They all pleasant and polite, with some degree of education, but staring at me, a bar-dancer. Look at me, shabby compared to your nice fellow students – oh, I'm such a terrible person!" (On the verge of tears.)

"Whoa, quit now!" (Pulls off the road, stops car, turns toward her,) "You're wrong! You're not a terrible person – erase that from your brain! You're just different. Sometimes it's good to be different. My friends were just a little surprised by your being different, but at the same time, I suspect, some admiring you for it or even becoming jealous. I think they found you attractive, too, especially the guys."

(She looks up at him, recovering slightly. He continues,) "I agree you need a little help with your appearance. I know you never had a mother to teach you stuff. Now, I have a favorite aunt here in town who runs a high-class salon-boutique. If you wish, you can go there for some advice and maybe clothes. She owes me a favor."

(New scene, next day. He, at home, on the phone with his aunt, split screen showing both,) "Well, hello to my favorite auntie, this is Roy."

"Why, Roy! 'Gooday', as the 'Aussies' say (there's one in my shop right now!) Oh, oh, I feel a request coming. What is it this time, favorite nephew?"

"I guarantee you're going to enjoy this, solving a special new problem

123

for me. By chance I met this girl, attractive basically, with a lot to her but kind of – what should I say – unpolished. She never had a mother to teach her the basics, if you know what I mean. I'd like you to help her in appearance and clothes. I can send her over if you agree. You may recall you owe me one."

(New scene – next evening. He sits in his living room, studying, quiet. She enters, has had a total appearance makeover; hair, face, clothing, shoes, accoutrements. He gasps seeing her, stares, speechless, drops his book, stunned! This scene continues silently awhile. Then she,) "And your aunt's not even through yet. I have to go back tomorrow. She's expecting some new clothes from Italy, says they'll be perfect for me. I think she really enjoyed doing this – worked all day on me, called in some colleagues for their opinions and suggestions." (Pause. He continues staring.) "You like it?"

(He finally arises, walks around her, looking up and down, then pronouncing the letters,) "O-M-G! O-M-G! I knew you were pretty underneath it all, but I didn't expect this. I don't know what to say except I'm glad I met you. And I surely will thank my wonderfully talented Auntie."

"You did all this. I'm so grateful. I think I felt inferior before, like I wasn't worth much in the big scheme of things. Now that's all changed. I feel so good. Maybe I can even become more of a person, study and learn some stuff, do something worthwhile."

(He takes both her hands, smiles, his face now close to hers, he staring into her eyes.

But then his doctor-to-be instinct takes over and he withdraws slightly,)

"Why, you only have one contact lens! Only in one eye!"

(She backs away a bit also, dejected,) "Wow, you surely know how to impress a girl! Mr. Romance himself! We're all alone, close together, you stare deeply into my eyes and then ask about my contact lens! I felt you were about to kiss me. Were you?"

"I was thinking about it."

"THINKING about it! Oh Dr. Grace, I need to give you an anatomy lesson! You have a brain to think with and a heart to feel with, both equally important, but you don't THINK about kissing a girl, you FEEL it. Oh, what they don't teach you in medical school!

But since you noticed, I'll let you in on a little secret – only my doctors and my mother, if she's still alive somewhere, know." (She removes the one contact and shows him her face. She now has one beautiful blue eye and one beautiful brown eye.

He stares at her closely, then steps back,) "I thought that was medically impossible!"

"My eye doctor said it's nearly impossible – 'anisocoria,' he called it. They're normal otherwise. It's actually kind of nice; if I want blue accents, I put a blue contact in the brown eye, and vice versa.

The other news is that I applied for the job of weather-girl at the local TV station, and have an audition day after tomorrow. I plan a lively performance, with some of my props from dance routines."

"That should be interesting!"

(New scene, interior of TV station two days later. Station manager, speaking in a hoarse voice on the telephone to "Al", the weather-reporter,) "You've got laryngitis too? Can't do the program today? No, I can't either. Lots of people have it, even the secretary is out. No, the techs can't. They have to run the electronics and cameras. We may have to cancel the weather report. What, two big weather fronts coming in? Wait, there's a girl coming in soon for an audition. You've interviewed her and like her? She's a "looker" with experience? She'll have to do it live!"

(New scene. Aida appears at the station, meets the station manager,) "Greetings, Sir. I'm here for the weather-reporter audition."

(Manager, continued rough voice,) "Come in. We've had a real problem here with our scheduled weather telecast for today. Both the regular reporter and I have laryngitis and can't go on camera. There are two big important weather fronts headed our way, so we can't cancel. Are you up to a live broadcast right away?"

"Sure. I'm a professional performer. No problem."

"Okay, let's rehearse the teleprompter so you're familiar with it. Air-time in twenty-minutes. You have an nine-minute sequence for your forecast."

"Fine, but let's teleprompter-practice for just a moment, then I'll need a few minutes for my own live-TV preparation."

(New scene. Aida in front of the TV camera; beautiful long wavy red hair, carefully-applied make-up and nail coloring, bright jewelry and accoutrements; dressed in a colorful, short, flouncy skirt; tight, pink camisole-style tee shirt with spaghetti shoulder straps and nothing underneath, plus a patterned shawl which partially covers her; and low-cut dance shoes without stockings. Behind her is a wall-size weather map with various symbols and lettering, computer-programmed to change appropriately throughout the forecast. The station manager is off to the side out of camera range, pointing to a large wall-clock as the second-hand approaches the vertical position. When it reaches exactly twelve, he gestures decisively to her as a signal to begin.)

"Good evening folks, or 'bon soir' as the French say. I'm Aida Saint Cyr, stand-in for 'Thunderstorm Al,' your regular weatherman, who has laryngitis and can't report this evening. And we have WILD news for you now. (She discards the shawl and throws shoulders back, marches boldly toward the camera,) two BIG FRONTS coming right at you tonight! The first with high winds, (she turns on a large floor fan, steps back, the "wind" blowing her skirt up high, revealing shapely legs and bikini panties. After a moment she turns off the fan,) "And then tomorrow morning comes the next: RAIN!" (She places a comic hat-like artificial flower on top of her head, holds a watering can over it, tilts the can, water flows over the "plant" and over her face and upper body, causing her wet tee shirt to cling even more tightly.) "But then comes a weather "INVERSION" That's where clouds turn UPSIDE DOWN!" (She performs a handstand against a post, part of the building structure off to the side and usually off camera, but not now. She is facing outward, feet and legs upward around it. Again her skirt falls over her face, an "R" rated momentary scene. She pulls up, using leg and abdominal muscles and then performs a brief "pole dance" as bar performers often do, twisting and waving arms. She next dismounts and puts on sun glasses,) "But soon, bright sun comes marching through. Don't forget to have a friend apply your sunblock." (She beckons one of the camera technicians with head-set and microphone, who comes near. She squeezes some sunblock onto his fingers, pulls down the front of her shirt a bit, he rubs it onto her upper chest, then,) "That's enough, Bob, I don't want to get all excited here on camera."

(Scene shifts to the darkened television monitor room, where the manager stands beside a technician who has his finger on a large electrical switch,) "This is pretty wild, boss. Should I cut to a commercial?"

"No. I may get fired for this, but keep it running."

(Scene back to Aida, live on camera,) "And after that, on Thursday afternoon, a sudden dust storm and everything turns brown." (She positions her face close up to the camera, closes her blue eye and points to the brown one. But then she opens her blue eye and points to it.) "But take heart! On Friday morning we have blue skies! But wait! Friday afternoon, ANOTHER front, wind and rain blowing us around AGAIN!" (She performs cartwheels across the studio-room, skirt flying, concluding in a floor-split, legs wide apart. She continues,) "And then a quiet weekend and I'll be worn out and sleep. Goodnight." (She spreads a bed-sheet on the floor, lies down on it, with eyes closed, snoring slightly.

Now to the monitor-room. The technician cuts to a commercial. Both he and the station manager staring at each other, wide-eyed, mouths open, speechless.)

(New scene: Next day, interior of the TV station, small conference table; station manager, Aida, and the regular weatherman, Al, sit soberly.)

Manager: "Well, now I have a tough decision to make. Al, you've been a good employee for us. But Aida, since your "Two-eyed girl's weather report," my phone's been ringing off the hook, companies and organizations all wanting to be sponsors for our weather reports. Your segment brought a huge positive response! Even the news media highlighted it. Al, I'd like to keep you, but I have to consider the economics."

Aida: "Sir, I've researched "Thunderstorm Al" on the internet. He's worked here for you over ten years with only a rare sick day. He's a family man, elder in his church, active in charities and leadership in both Boy and Girl Scouts.

Sir, I'm making your decision easy. I'm withdrawing my application – want to go to school anyway. I hope you keep him and even consider a raise."

(Later. Roy speaking as narrator, with action as described depicted on screen, similar to earlier in the script,) "We soon married and she helped me finish medical school. She had her fallopian tubes surgically 'untied' and then delivered us beautiful twins, a blue-eyed boy and a brown-eyed girl, both with red hair.

I considered specialty training in obstetrics-gynecology, though she questioned this."

Aida: "Why would you want to spend your days staring at – what should I say? – female, er, anatomy?"

Roy: "You may think it's like that but it's not. It's the one specialty, as opposed to general family practice, that includes a whole spectrum of specialties: surgery; internal medicine with such subsets as endocrinology, infectious disease, and cancer; even aspects of psychiatry, since many women tend to tell all their secrets, no matter how deeply hidden, to their gynecologists. It's full of drama, not to mention science and compassion. Of course the patient population is limited to women, but that's okay."

Narrator: "I went on to post-graduate training in that specialty of "OB-GYN", then choosing an academic career, stayed on at the medical school in a junior-faculty position as Instructor.

She went to school, obtained a degree in Philosophy with minor in Education, then a job as grade-school teacher with occasional substitute fill-in as television weather-reporter (dressing and behaving conservatively!) As an avocation, she successfully wrote children's books.

But every year, on a certain anniversary date, we invited friends and family to our home, drank champagne and once again played the video-recording of that notorious, that hilarious, that absolutely unique 'Two-Eyed Girl's Weather Report!' "

(Her "report" replays on the screen, followed by, "The End". But then, after several seconds, that phrase is replaced on the screen by, "BUT WAIT! …not yet…")

A Sequel

Brief explanatory notation on the screen: "Several years later, the twins now three years old; a Saturday late afternoon, the family at home, relaxing in their den."

Action then resumes:

The door-bell rings.

The twins run to answer it.

At the door stands an elderly woman, nicely dressed, carrying only a small purse; a slight smile.

The twins race back inside, "Mom, Dad, there's someone here!"

(Aida comes to the door, a slight frown, squints her eyes,) "Yes?"

(The lady, eyes moist, emotional, speaks haltingly,) "It took me a long time to find you. First your name change, then again to a married name, plus moving around, widely different locations and jobs. Later I hired a private detective and she finally was able to trace you here."

(Aida – amazed, now wide-eyed, staring,) "M-m-mother? Mother? Is that you?"

(Momentary silence. Shock. Almost disbelief. Roy and the twins approach from behind. Both women now openly in tears and embracing warmly.

Mother, backing away slightly,) "I have an apology to offer and a story to tell."

Aida: "No apology needed – and I have a story to tell also. Come in."

THE…actual… END

Screenplay – Prologue
(Precedes title-screen)

(Background music, soft, played by a high-school marching band, mildly discordant and off-key, mutes during spoken lines, then resumes during title and introductory screens. It ceases when action begins again after the opening sequences, recurring as noted in the script.)

Opening scene: Camera focuses in on an interior wood and opaque-glass door labeled "Central High School – Faculty Lounge."

Scene shifts inside; morning sunlight streams in from several windows; visible through them are outside walkways leading up to the building. Flowers and foliage suggest spring. Small groups of students are walking toward the entrance.

Inside the lounge several faculty members are reading newspapers, relaxing, drinking coffee. A background wall-clock shows seven-thirty.

(First teacher (FT), male, sitting at a small table, to football coach (HC), standing,) "Mornin', Coach. How goes it?"

(HC) "Oh, you know, same-ol', same-ol'." (Walks on by, sipping coffee.)

(Second teacher (ST), male, seated, reading newspaper,) "Hey, listen to this! Miss Hatfield died! You remember, she was that great old gal who ran a small private charity-type school near here. Says its formal name was 'Miss Hatfield's School for the Talented but Socially Disadvantaged.'" (Continues reading,) "Long ago as a young adult, she was a budding concert-violinist when her fiancé, a Marine, was killed in the war. She then abruptly gave up the stage, shunned society and devoted the entire remainder of her long life to the school. She never married. Her current students will be reassigned to various public institutions here in the city."

(FT, looking out of the window, pause, now staring, speaking excitedly,) "Oh my, and here come three of them on the sidewalk right now! Let's see – a girl in a wheelchair, holding a violin case, with a black fellow pushing her, and then – what? Maybe a native-American Indian-looking guy behind them. "

(ST, now staring out also, slight pause,) "Wow! I have this strange feeling that our Central High School will never be quite the same again."

(FT, studying the three,) "Hmm, I believe you may be right."

MISS HATFIELD'S SCHOOL

(Sometimes Titled "Trio" or "Heritage")

– screenplay–

An epic film of: suffering, humiliation, courage, betrayal, jealousy, dedication, endurance, awakening, lust, redemption, failure and eventual triumph –
– All the usual stuff –

Title-character based on a true individual, now deceased; a distant-relative of the author.

(transient screen)

"Knowledge, Compassion, Physical Strength, an Appreciation of Beauty. These are the four cornerstones upon which a noble and enduring character can be formed: Yea, indeed, upon which even a great and lasting civilization may be built."
— Ancient Greek aphorism.*

* One of those "antiquarians" must have said something to this effect – after all, those guys were pretty smart!

(Secondary-title screen, then resumption of action. Background music stops.)

— The Artist --

(Scene – close-up of black former Hatfield-student (AS)'s bare arm, with medical tourniquet above the elbow, causing the superficial veins to expand. A full syringe with needle, held by a pair of hands, is poised to pierce the vein for a drug injection. The arm quivers in fear. Camera backs away slowly, showing AS seated in a wooden chair, arm extended over a small table, all within a poorly-lit, barely furnished room, a single light bulb dangling above. In addition to AS, two nicely dressed young black males (B1 and B2) sit at the table, B1 holding the syringe expectantly. AS's face sweats, his expression reflecting anxiety, grimacing. B1 and B2 are calm, soft-talking.)

(B1) "Easy now. You'll soothe way-down once this 'goody-juice' circulates. You'll be really happy then! Remember those glad times we had before that witch, Hatfield, kidnapped you? Recall the dreams? Ecstasy? Floating through clouds without a care! Well, we're all back now, that bitch is gone forever, dead. No one to stand between us anymore. I've even got some fine jobs lined up for you to pull off, to get the big bills we'll need for some really great joy-juice. Nobody to keep you jailed-up, away from us anymore!" (Pause, B1 continues) "So here we go into that nice vein, just waiting for happiness."

(Camera again focuses on AS's arm, as B1 starts to advance the syringe and needle forward. Camera then backs away showing AS sweating profusely and extremely anxious. He suddenly bolts up and tears off his tourniquet, shouting,) "No! No! I am free! Now I'm free and I'll stay free! I won't go under again!"

(AS runs toward the door. B2 draws a hand-gun from his belt and starts up after him. B1, laughing evilly, restrains B2 and commands,) "Let him go! He's nuts. There's plenty of others." (B2 stops, sits back down and replacing the hand-gun in his belt, laughs also.)

(New scene – Interior door with metal plaque inscribed "Central High School Award-Winning Graphic Arts Department -- Classroom Studio" Camera withdraws slightly, showing AS anxious and sweating, racing from outside toward the door. He bolts through it noisily. The camera follows him inside where numerous students, mostly female, sit at individual small easels painting quietly. They pause and stare at his loud entry.

The art teacher (TA), middle-aged African-American standing among the students, looks at her watch and then at AS, frowning, admonishes,) "I know you've just transferred in from another school, but really, we do expect you in class on time."

(AS, still anxious,) "Sorry, Ma'am. Sorry."

(The camera follows him as he hurries to his own easel, which has been placed a slight distance from the others and has been turned with the painting-side facing a window, its image thus hidden from the remaining class's view. His canvas and tray of paints and brushes are significantly larger than those of the other students. He throws back the sheet covering his work and after only a brief study of its image, begins to apply paints in sweeping, bold moves, still anxious and breathing hard.

Camera shifts over to TA, moving slowly among the students who are methodically reproducing landscapes from photographs onto their small canvases. She offers brief suggestions and comments while studying their individual works. Reaching AS, she is startled -- a small gasp, eyes widened, backs off,) "What's this?" (Pause, staring at the painting, which is pure abstraction, in brilliant colors, convoluted shapes, arresting and emotional to the observer's eye.) "The assignment was for landscape."

(AS, not slowing his work even as he speaks,) "This is a landscape, the landscape of my mind. I've never been outside the city here, never seen a forest or mountain. Saw some trees behind the city dump once, by where I used to live. But I imagine what it must feel like to see 'em, to experience nature. 'Scapes don't always just have to be outdoors, trees and grass. They can be distantly-viewed vistas of anything, real or imagined, perceived through the senses or merely felt emotionally."

(TA, frowning, surprised,) "And where did you get such a large canvas?"

(AS, continuing to paint,) "I brought my own over from Miss Hatfield's. She always encouraged me to paint. I set it up here, to catch the sunlight through the window. It bolds the colors, don't you think?"

(TA studies AS and his painting, viewing it from multiple angles and perspectives as AS continues to work rapidly. She develops a slight frown, then walks over to the Art Department Director (AD), an older black male who is chatting with one of the other students.)

(AD, looking up,) "What's wrong? You seem upset."

(TA) "Come over here a moment, please. Let me show you the work of one of our new students."

(They proceed over to AS. AD smiles, nods a greeting, studies the work, frowns, then appears more deeply concerned. Pause.)

(AD) "You did this?"

(AS continues to paint rapidly even as he replies,) "Yes, Sir. Not finished yet, though I stayed late yesterday to work on it."

(AD continues to stare at the canvas from various vantage points. Pause.)

(AD) "How old are you?"

(AS) "Seventeen, Sir." (Pause) "And most of those seventeen were pretty ragged. Sometimes I feel more like seventy-seven!"

(AD glances knowingly at TA, then,) "Come, both of you please, to my office for a few minutes."

(Scene shifts to his small office. AD sits on his desk, TA standing nearby. He gestures to AS to have a seat.)

(AS) "No thanks. If it's okay, Sir, I do better standing." (Still tense)

(AD, concerned,) "That's quite a work of art you're creating out there. Tell me a little about yourself. I understand you just transferred in from Miss Hatfield's School ."

(AS) "I don't do well with words, Sir, particularly about myself. I'm better at expressing with paints – with colors, lines, shapes, tones, hues." (His facial expression is one of intensity. He gestures freely with hands and arms, intermittently making fists while talking about his art,) "I have these feelings, Sir, these emotions. They come out so freely in my work, but they defy words. I can tell you that Miss Hatfield rescued me from the Project, gave me a place to live, encouraged me to paint. "

(AD) "Do you have a place to live, now that she has died?

(AS) "I'll have to move out. No place to go."

(Pause. TA and AD continue to study him silently. AS's facial expression is now one of sadness. As he reflects on his situation, this changes to one of fear, then wide-eyed to a near-hysterical outburst,) "NO – NO – PLEASE DON'T SEND ME BACK TO THE PROJECT! I'll do anything! I promise never to be late again!" (Fists clenched; near tears,) "They'll kill me!" (In desperation, he turns, grasps TA's forearms harshly, then realizing this inappropriate, he releases them, his tone softening, "I'm sorry Ma'am. Please forgive me."

(TA and AD are greatly moved by his plea and the emotional scene unfolding before them).

(TA takes both his hands, speaks firmly, warmly,) "Listen to me. No one is sending you back to the Project. It's okay. You're among people who understand. You have an obvious very special talent and we will help you develop it." (She releases his hands, but AD notices his bare forearm and lifts it into view. All three stare at the needle marks.)

(AD, comforting,) "I know what you're going through. We can help." (Pause, releases his arm.) "My wife and I have an empty garage apartment. You can stay there for now. Come back here after class and we'll arrange it."

(AS) "Yes, Sir."

(AD) "We'll work with you. I believe you're extremely gifted in addition to being very courageous."

(AS has softened, still serious, shakes hands with TA and AD,) "Thank you. You're both so kind. God will bless you, and someday, God willing, I'll repay you." (Pause) "May I go back to my work now?"

(Scene ends.)

(Secondary Title Screen followed by resumption of action)

— The Athlete —

(Scene: high school classroom, students at small tables, the teacher (AT) at the head of class with desk and blackboard. She is young, animated, pretty; plainly dressed with no jewelry. The American-Indian former Hatfield student (IS) stands beside his table, simply-dressed in slightly over-sized clothes which tend to hide his muscular athletic body.)

(AT) "And so we welcome our new transfer student – welcome to ALGEBRA, THE BEST CLASS AT CENTRAL HIGH!" (Pumps fist for emphasis. Students respond with claps, cheers, foot-stomping. AT lifts hands, palms forward, eyes closed in a gesture for silence. Noise abates. She continues to address IS,) "You may be seated." (IS takes his place at the table. AT, smiling at him,) "Now I know a mid-semester change is difficult, so anything at all I can do for you, just let me know." (Soft whistles, "Woo!" and "Whee!" sounds erupt from male students. AT slams a book down on her desk, proclaiming loudly,) "Now stop that!" (Noise ceases.) "So to get on with Algebra: remember, 'X' represents the unknown quantity. First you construct a numerical equation, which is like a set of scales with equal amounts on each side, that is, balanced. (She draws a set of scales on the blackboard, "X+A" on one side and a box marked "BxC" on the other side.) "We'll let 'A, B and C' mean 'known numbers.' Then we do the exact same mathematical thing to each side of the scale to keep it balanced, until you have 'X' alone on one side and a known value on the other side, and, 'voila,' you've solved for 'X'."

(As she was speaking, the camera shifted from her at the blackboard over to IS' face, showing him staring at her. Camera then shifts back to her lecturing, now wearing only a bra and panties. The camera once more to him; he blinks his eyes repeatedly, slapping his own cheek. Camera again to her, lecturing, now fully clothed. She interrupts her instruction, walks toward him with a slight frown,) "Are you alright?"

(IS, now behaving normally,) "Yes, Miss, sorry. Okay now."

(New scene: high school football locker-room. Lighting is dim, somewhat concealing IS's taut muscular physique. He is dressed in athletic shorts and tee-shirt, attempting to put on shoulder pads, having mild difficulty. Speaks to another student-athlete (SA),) "I'm new at this, just now came out for spring practice, a little late, can you help me adjust these?"

(SA, assisting with the pads,) "Never played football before? Well,

137

'good luck' is all I can say."

(IS) "Thanks. I have a strange feeling I'll need it. "

(Scene – early dawn, barely light, high school football practice field with small bleachers, empty except for former coach (FC), age forties, sitting in a lower-row, partially reclining, hand on chin, a distant look on his face, a walking-cane nearby. Pause. Silence. Then he is startled by IS entering the track in front of the bleachers through a nearby gate. IS, sweating from running, is dressed in athletic shorts and shoes, wearing football shoulder-pads under a faded grey jersey. He removes the jersey and with mild difficulty, the pads; a tee-shirt remains. Now for the first time, obvious to the viewer is his trim, powerful body. He sets the pads on a lower bench and begins a stretching routine, notices FC observing him, nods,) "Mornin'."

(FC) "Mornin'." (Pause. He rises and walking with the cane, approaches IS,) "Haven't seen you around here before."

(IS, continues stretching,) "No, Sir, new here – transferred over to Central High from a small private school, so I've had to change location for my morning workouts. Also, 'been wearing those pads some, to get used to 'em. 'Gone out for spring practice to get a feel for team sports."

(FC, showing interest,) "Morning workouts?"

(IS) "Yeah, always have. I've got this thing about the human body. Almost like a religion with me. Pretty amazing." (Continues working various muscle groups.)

(FC) "I know what you mean. I was a coach all my life, 'til this happened," (points to lame leg,) "then they put me out to pasture. I come out here early some days, recall years past, happier times. "

(IS, stops stretching, studies FC,) "I'm sorry."

(FC, eyes downcast, sighs,) "It's okay. I'm making it." (He brightens somewhat,) "So what's your routine?"

(IS, also cheerful now,) "Three mornings a week I run 'couple of miles to a track, this one now, some fifty- and hundred-yard sprints, run home again. Mixed weight-lifting, rope-jumping and bag-punching once a week, swim laps one morning, a nice long bicycle ride Sundays. On Saturdays – you'll laugh when I tell you about Saturdays."

(FC, showing more interest,) "What?"

(IS, smiling,) "I dance! I work part-time over at the Rehabilitation Hospital, and we have a dance instructor nine-to-one Saturdays, to help the patients. They love it. The ones that are able move around to the music, and those in wheelchairs smile and tap their fingers. They look forward to it all week – has even sparked a few romances among patients out there on the dance-floor. I help the instructor and have gotten so good I'm actually her assistant now."

(FC, smiles,) "Hey, I'm not laughing! Dance is really helpful for rhythm and coordination. Back when I was football coach, we had a professional teacher. I'd show the team a film-clip of some great old dancer like Fred Astaire, then I'd show 'em one of a ball carrier 'dancing' through a pack of would-be tacklers. They got the idea real quick. Even those big muscular line-men benefited." (Pause) "So where'd you learn to do all this? That's a mighty impressive routine."

(IS) "I have a friend who was a multi-sport player awhile back, named Royal Grace. Every time he comes back through town he helps me, particularly weights and swimming. I do the running pretty much on my own."

(FC, excitedly,) " Roy Grace! An outstanding high school champ. I coached him on this very field." (Points. Pause. Studies IS,) "Okay, let's see you do some stuff."

(IS, enthusiastically,) "Yes, Sir!"

(FC pauses, looks up and down the running track,) "First, I want you to get back there thirty yards or so to that post," (Points,) "and then skip, just like little kids do, up to this finish-line here. (Points in front of them to the track.)

(IS does so while FC watches carefully. He returns to FC, again expectantly.)

(FC) "Now I want you back there again, but run backward to here."

(IS performs as directed, while FC observes closely.)

(FC, becoming excited.) "Okay, now run one lap on this quarter-mile track. Start out, up to that far turn, just coasting along, slow, but soft and even. Then on the backstretch, pick it up to about a two-mile pace, moderately long strides, arms smooth. Now, on this home-stretch I want you to give it every possible ounce of speed you have, as if the very devil was chasing you!"

(IS runs the lap at the three speeds described. FC follows the action intently. IS returns to FC, panting and sweating. Hopeful.)

(FC, now somewhat emotional, walks with his cane around IS, studying him. Pause, then speaking softly,) "Okay. We can do it. We can do it."

(IS, puzzled, now recovered,) "Do what, Sir?"

(FC, excitedly,) "You give me forty-minutes here three mornings a week for the next three weeks. We can win the hundred-yard dash at the State High School Spring Open Track Meet!"

(IS, wide-eyed, surprised, stares at FC.)

(FC) "You've great coordination and a natural, animal-like fluid motion. But we need to work on your elbows and neck!"

(IS, puzzled,) "Elbows? Neck?"

(FC) "Remember, you run with every cell in your body, from scalp to toes – more than that – to the soles of your shoes. Which reminds me, we need to get you different shoes."

(Pause. FC and IS stand staring at each other, wide smiles. FC extends his hand,) "'Deal?"

(IS extends his,) "'Deal!" (They shake hands.)

(FC walks away rapidly with his cane, talking loudly over his shoulder, "Same time, day after tomorrow."

(IS) "Wait! Sir, I didn't get your name – "

(FC) "Details later. We've work to do!"

(New scene: high-school football locker-room, now pre-game, IS in front of the uniform-distribution counter. Attendant hands IS a red game jersey.)

(Attendant) "Sorry, it's the last one I have. You'll have to be number zero."

(IS, sighing,) "That's okay. Zero is better than nothing." (Takes jersey.)

(Other student-athlete (SA), close-by,) "'Zero is better than nothing!' That's kind of philosophical. Wonder what our algebra teacher would say about that."

(IS, smiling, speaks dreamily, eyes half-closed,) "Algebra teacher. Algebra teacher. Oh, wow. I dream about her."

(SA) "You and a couple-dozen other guys."

(New scene: high school football stadium filled with fans, night game, bright lights, marching band seated at lower levels providing background music, loud, energetic and somewhat discordant, as camera sweeps slowly about this grand scene. After a short interval of time, a radio announcer (RA)'s voice is heard and band music attenuates as camera continues slow sweep.)

(RA) "Yes, ladies and gentlemen, football fans state-wide! This is THE spring high-school sports event we have all been waiting for."

(Camera now focuses in on RA, seated in front of his microphone, other media personnel close-by in a small upper-level press booth. RA continues,) "As most of you know, this annual contest is the culmination of Central High's football spring training program. Through the years this

140

traditional intra-squad game has grown in stature and popularity 'til it even rivals the regular fall season! Our head coach, beloved by players and fans alike, gets the credit for developing this exciting annual contest. The main difference from other schools' events is that our graduating seniors participate in the full spring practice and of course will play here tonight. This innovation by our coach some years ago serves two needs: first, some of our seniors go right into college ball, and we all want them to be ready, in top shape. Also, those graduating are encouraged to pass on their skills and help the underclassmen, who will comprise the regular fall team – help them play their best for GOOD OLD CENTRAL HIGH!

Now the way it works is this: the assistant coach and his tonight-rival, the head coach, have chosen players alternately for their respective teams, the Blues and the Reds. The assistant coach traditionally gets to pick first, and guess who he chose? You're right! The senior number-one high school athlete in the state, and I don't even need to tell you his name. A multi-sport star ever since freshman year. Just one of his claims to fame: he set a record in the hundred-yard dash only last fall." (Pause) "And here he comes now, leading the blue team onto the field, appropriately wearing number one on his jersey!"

(Thunderous ovation as cheerleaders, followed by "number-one" (NO) and his team in blue uniforms, stream out of the gate, running under the goal post and onto the playing field. Applause attenuates significantly and the band music is more clearly heard as a similar entrance by the red team occurs at the opposite end of the field; IS, wearing number zero on his red jersey, brings up the rear.

Longer pause indicating passage of time, screen blanks momentarily, new scene: camera focuses on scoreboard, showing five minutes remaining in the first quarter of play, score Blues twenty-one, Reds zero.

Camera shifts to the head coach (HC), pacing the side-line in front of his red-clad players seated on the bench. He is age-thirties, dressed with coat and tie, a baseball cap. He tends to be emotional and overly dramatic in voice, posturing and gestures. Episodic background cheers and band music continue. He grimaces as he looks at the play action, sporadically covering his eyes in dismay, looks up at the scoreboard, groans.

IS arises from the bench holding his helmet, approaches HC.)

(IS) "Sir -- "

(HC, still looking at play-action, moans again, grimacing, shakes head in disbelief. Glances only briefly at IS,) "Yeah, whadayou want? – Oh! – Ouch!"

(IS) "Sir, I'd like to go into the game."

(HC, continues his painful play action observation,) "Any reason I should put you in?"

(IS) "I have a pretty good body."

(HC, over-reacting, gesturing wildly,) "Oh, spare me! Spare me! A good body! Now I've heard everything! Why-oh-why did I ever become a football coach! Why didn't I become a nice dentist like my dear departed mother wanted." (Gazes heaven-ward, palms together in prayer-fashion, then crosses himself as a Roman Catholic,) "Sure there are some cheerleaders out there with pretty good bodies!" (Stares into the camera,) "Actually they'd probably do better out on the field than those red guys!" (Pause, shouting toward the play-action, making a sign of "T" with hands,) "Time-out! Time-out!" (Then over his shoulder to IS,) "Okay Mister Goodbody, go in for –" (Muffled. IS dons helmet, runs onto the field, replacing another red player; all are discussing strategy during brief time-out.)

(IS addresses team-mate SA,) "Hey, tell me, -- I'm still learning the rules of this game – but I've noticed that blue guy with number one on his jersey, boy, he's good, but when he's running with the ball, just as he crosses the scrimmage line, he's not holding it too tightly. So I wanted to ask about the rules. If I pull the ball away from him before the referee's whistle blows, can I run for a touchdown?"

(SA, starts to chuckle,) "Sure, sure, you're going to take the ball away from the best athlete in the state, sure, then run for a touchdown – " (Chuckles grow into full-grown laughter, then a hysterical outburst.

Camera shifts back to RA in press-box.)

(RA) "Pretty one-sided game here, folks. The assistant-coach's blue guys running rampant in the first quarter of play. Twenty-one zero and they are already down to the Red twenty-yard line, ready to score again. (Pause) Time-out now up." (Pause) "Wait a minute – what is this? Referee signaling delay-of-game penalty? Looks like an injury, red player down. I don't understand – during time out? Let's look through the ol' binoculars, see if we can tell what the heck is going on there on the field."

(Pause, RA peers through large binoculars, other reporters also surprised, pointing, mumbling. RA continues excitedly,) "Ladies and gentlemen, for all my years of high-school sports broadcasting, this is a new one on me! Listen to this – delay of game caused by a player lying on the ground, laughing hysterically! He can't stop! Absolutely amazing."

(Pause, new scene, football play-action resumes. Slow-motion filming now with sound muted for this sequence, camera focuses close-up. Blue team on offense, quarterback under center, NO in tailback position.

Quarterback takes the snap, hands the ball off to NO charging through center of the line. IS in defensive line-backer position, sinks a shoulder into NO, wrestles the football from his grip, then sprints onward carrying the ball. NO recovers his balance and races in pursuit, but IS has had several yards head-start. Camera, still in slow-motion, backs away from above, showing the two opposing players speeding downfield, IS gradually lengthening his lead over NO. Camera shifts back to RA in the press-booth, now no longer slow motion. RA wide-eyed and speaking excitedly into the microphone,) "Yes, fans, he stole the ball from Blue number-one and is now racing hell-bent for the goal line! But who is that Red player? Number zero – " (Looks at his program,) "He's not even listed on the player roster, and, I can't believe it, he's PULLING AWAY from Blue number-one, pulling away from the fastest sprinter in the state! " (Pause, listening briefly to another reporter,) "Someone says his name is 'Goodbody,' and he's outrunning our speediest racer!" (Other reporters in the press box standing, pointing, excited. Camera now back to play action, IS crosses the goal line untouched. RA continues shouting,) "And he scores! Red touchdown!" (Crowd roars, loud applause, band plays discordantly. Camera shifts back to HC, overjoyed, shouting, jumping – removes his cap and throws it wildly onto the ground. He grabs one of his sideline players and pointing on-field, instructs,) "Quick, go in, tell 'em to RUN for two points after touchdown – NOT to kick – give the ball to THAT GUY! 'ZERO'! Straight up the middle!"

(Pause, again slow-motion filming of play action, now with intermittent freeze-frame sequencing to enhance clarity. Sound totally muted. This scene is dramatically intense and must be staged carefully.

Red team's ball at point-after-touchdown play. The ball is snapped to the quarterback; he hands off to IS charging the middle line. IS dances, cuts, avoids tacklers initially, then as they cling onto him, he crosses the goal line dragging them and falls; the referee signals "score" and his whistle momentarily breaks the film's silence. NO is the opposing line-backer and is close by. A very brief but definite, obvious, time-interval after the referee's whistle blows, the camera focusing on NO's face showing rage, then quickly backing off to show the action: NO dives shoulder-first onto the fallen IS, striking him on the lower leg. A cracking sound transiently breaks the muted silence. IS reflexively throws his head back violently, his helmet flying loose and off. Continued slow motion and silence, camera now focuses on IS's face and upper body. He grimaces in pain, eyes tightly shut, he is collapsed on the turf, bites into his own bare forearm in anguish, tears flow down over the arm, mix with blood from the bite and drip onto

143

the ground. The film's subscript reveals his silent plea, "Spirit of my father, comfort me at this time. Spirit of my mother, stay close." Camera backs away from above, slowly at first, then rapidly, continued slow-motion filming and silence, though freeze-frame sequencing ceases.

An ambulance pulls onto the playing field and attendants carefully load IS onto a stretcher and into the vehicle. Camera fades.

New scene: IS alone, lying in a hospital bed, facing right, head of the bed rolled up, left lower leg in a cast which rests elevated on pillows. Morning sun streams through the window. Silence. Camera closes in on IS's face and upper body, his expression reflecting a somber mood. He speaks aloud to himself in a form of soliloquy, though not looking at the camera. Sighs, then thoughtfully, pausing between comments,) "Oh, boy." "First Miss Hatfield dies." "She was all I had." "Now this." (Regards his casted leg. Sighs,) "You do the best you can. You keep on going and you do the best that you can. That's all I know to do." (Pause. A knock on the door.) "Yes?" (Two coaches, FC, with walking cane, and HC enter. IS smiles and greets them,) "Good morning, Coaches – nice to see you both! Come on in."

(HC, tending to the dramatic as always, smiling, starts in but then spotting the injured leg on pillows, stops abruptly, wide-eyed, sudden worried facial appearance, steps back, arms outstretched stopping FC, speaks anxiously,) "Gee, Kid, are you okay?"

(IS) "Well, I feel fine, but as you can see, I won't be running races anytime soon."

(HC) "I mean, no pain?"

(IS) "None."

(HC) "They taking care of you – I mean, food and stuff?"

(IS) "Yep, fine. The food is actually pretty good here."

(HC, now smiles slightly, approaches IS,) "Well, I'm glad of that."

(FC) "Yeah, you look okay except for that leg."

(HC, now happy and excited, talking rapidly, animated,) "Well, kid, do you know what you did last night?"

(IS) "Sure do, broke my leg!"

(HC) "No, no – before that!"

(IS grimaces slightly, touches forehead with a finger,) "That part is kind of fuzzy."

(HC) "Have you seen today's newspapers and TV?"

(IS) "No."

(Now both coaches are quite excited, talking loudly and rapidly,

144

speaking alternately,) "Well kid, let me tell you!" "The whole state is talking about you!" "Headlines on the sports page!"

(HC) "My phone 'been ringing off the hook! College scouts, TV stations, sports-writers, all wanting to know who the heck you are!"

(FC) "Nobody knew your name!"

(HC) "Someone thought your name was 'Goodbody.'"

(FC) "They call you the 'zero-hero' because of your jersey number."

(IS) "What?"

(HC & FC) "YOU OUTRAN THE FASTEST SPRINTER IN THE STATE!"

(IS) "Really?"

(FC) "You even inspired the red team to win, thirty-six to twenty-one!"

(IS) "Wow!"

(HC) "Who taught you to run like that?"

(IS, pointing to FC,) "This fine coach right here."

(HC, looking at FC,) "You did that?"

(IS, interrupting,) "He surely did, and in a very short period of time, too."

(FC, demurely,) "The lad was a pleasure to work with."

(Pause. HC steps back, studies FC, develops a slight frown,) "You're really getting around pretty well with that cane."

(FC) "Improvin'. Goin' to physical therapy sessions. Those guys know their stuff."

(Pause, HC speaking to FC in a serious tone,) "We've got to get you back to full-time coaching."

(FC, visibly affected, startled,) "You mean that?"

(HC) "Sure do. Actually I've got an opening right now. You call me in the morning and we'll work it out."

(FC, emotional,) "I'll do that – yes, Sir, yes Sir." (Then covering up for his moistening eyes, wipes his nose with a handkerchief, speaking softly,) "Darn allergies acting up."

(Pause, a knock on door, IS answers,) "Come in." (Medical Doctor (MD) enters, holding an x-ray. He is forties-age, dressed in green surgical scrub clothes and long white coat, accompanied by a student and a female nurse (FN) carrying a patient chart.)

(IS) "Good morning,` Doctor. " (They shake hands) "Know these two coaches?"

(MD, shaking hands with HC and FC,) "Sure do. They send me some business over the years – like right now." (points to IS,) "Mornin', gents.

And this is our faithful orthopedic-specialist nurse, Ms. J. J. Jones. Our docs' saying is, 'If J.J. doesn't know the answer, then the question's not worth asking.' And our medical student on surgery rotation." (They smile and nod greetings.)

(HC) "Do you want us to leave?"

(MD) "No. You may be interested in this."

(MD faces IS,) "Now to go over things from the start, as I know last night you might not have understood."

(MD holds up x-ray to the light, points,) "The bad news is: this long bone in your left lower-leg is broken, the thin outer bone called the 'fibula' by us docs, that goes from the knee down to the ankle. But, now hear this, the good news is: it's what we describe as a 'simple fracture', meaning no displacement of the bone or damage to other structures like joints, nerves, et cetera. So, it will heal completely, but you have to be patient. We're talking a couple' months total. We'll get you into a walking-cast in two weeks, which will make life a whole lot easier. Then by late summer you'll be good as new, and I'll bet these two coaches have some plans for you by then." (indicates HC and FC).

(HC, excitedly,) "We sure do!"

(FC) "You can get an athletic college scholarship for sure!"

(HC) "Do you know what you want to be when you grow up? What you want to study?"

(FC, laughing,) "Grow up? Looks to me like he's pretty well grown."

(HC, smiling,) "You're right there, Coach."

(IS) "Well, I'm almost afraid to say it, but I have always dreamed of becoming a medical doctor someday," (eyes downcast,) "but I have no money or help."

(MD, holding hands up in gesture,) "Wait, there are med-school assistance programs and scholarships – do you make good grades?"

(IS) "Oh, I love to study, learn stuff. Straight A's. Miss Hatfield was forever amazed."

(MD) "Okay. I can show you how to do it later, how to apply to medical school later in college."

(Medical Student,) "And I'll come visit another day and tell you all about it."

(IS, beaming,) "Wow! Totally awesome! You think there's even a chance I could become an orthopedic surgeon like you, and help those terribly injured patients?"

(MD) "I don't see why not. Many doctor-former-athletes choose orthopedics."

(Camera focuses in on IS's wide-eyed happy face, then fades to new scene.)

(Scene: IS now alone in his room, staring ahead, speaks aloud,) "An MD! I'm going to do it. I'll do it!" (Interrupted by a knock on his door,) "Come in."

(Student athlete "number one" (NO) enters, hesitantly, meekly, speaks softly,) "Okay to come in? I know you hate me."

(IS, puzzled,) "What? What's going on?"

(NO) "D'you know who I am?"

(IS, studies him,) "No." (pause,) "Wait, I think so – the other team – hey! Great athlete! Thanks for coming by."

(NO) "No, you don't understand – I'm the guy that hit you on the leg – I didn't – I mean, I was angry – I – "

(IS, interrupting,) "Hey, no, say no more! Stuff happens."

(NO, interrupting also,) "Wait, I want to – "

(IS) "Stop! I won't hear it. That's all past. We have to get on with things, the future. What's-to-come is all that counts."

(NO) "Okay." (Pause,) "That's kind of you." (For the first time, NO looks at IS carefully,) "Are you okay, I mean, taken care of 'n everything?"

(IS) "Yes, okay, good care. The doc says after a few months I'll be totally normal; he'll get me up walking in two weeks."

(NO) "Surely glad to hear that. Seems like you're doing fairly well, all considered."

(NO looks about the room, notices furniture and wall art,) "Wow, pretty 'homey' type room for a hospital."

(IS, leans forward,) "Ha, ha, I'll tell you a little secret. Did you notice how I'm in a different part of the hospital from the regular patient wards?"

(NO) "Yeah, way around in the back of the hospital."

(IS) "Not many people know this, but I live here, full time."

(NO, puzzled,) "What?"

(IS) "It's kind of a long story. You see, I was an orphan, or what used to be called a 'foundling' in old times. As a baby I was literally left on Miss Hatfield's doorstep, with no traceable parents, and she raised me. I mean, I have no family or possessions or stuff like that. She found this room for me awhile back. I do some odd jobs around the hospital, mow the lawn, a little of this and that. In return they give me this room, meals in their cafeteria and a little pocket money, plus I get to use their big gym and pool. (Pause. NO regards IS sympathetically. IS continues on,) "Wait, I do have one possession, and I'll show it to you. No one else except Miss Hatfield has ever

147

seen it. Look there under my clothes in that second drawer." (Points. NO extracts an envelope and hands it to IS, who removes a discolored sheet of paper, carefully unfolds it, hands it to NO.)

(NO reads aloud the scrawled writing slowly, movingly,) "'Dear Miss Hatfield, I have heard you are a kind woman and help people in trouble. Please take my son. I am dying and can no longer care for him. His father was American Indian, Hopi Tribe, and loved nature. May God bless you. May God protect this child. – His Mother.'" (NO folds the letter, hands it back to IS,) "Jeez, I mean, I'm sorry, you weren't old enough to know your mother?"

(IS) "Funny you should ask that. 'Know how some mothers hum little tunes when they tend their babies? I think somewhere in the back of my memory I must remember that. Sometimes when I run, 'specially in the first warm dawns of spring, I'm sure I hear her humming – her arms seem around me. And in the cool mornings of fall, running in forest paths, I feel the strength of my father. Strange, my contact to them – I can almost see them."

(NO, emotional,) "Wow, that's harsh." (Pause) "Is there anything I can do for you?"

(Pause, IS reflecting, smiles,) "Well, actually, yes. I have few friends since Miss Hatfield's students are mostly gone. It would be great if you and I could be buddies. We both share the athletic-scene pretty strongly."

(NO, covering up for his moistening eyes,) "Excuse me just a moment while I borrow your bathroom." (NO exits to bathroom, turns on sink faucet to provide cover-noise, stares at himself in the mirror, speaks out loud,) "Jesus! This guy has nothing! He lives alone up here in this room like a God-blessed saint. And then I hurt him, purposefully, injure him. What kind of a person does that make me?" (Pause) "And then he asks for my friendship. Jeez, this is like the Bible, or opera, or something." (Pause, rinses face, stares again at himself, speaks resolutely,) "Okay now, pull yourself together and do the right thing." (Exits to bedroom.)

(IS) "You okay?"

(NO, smiling) "Yeah." (Pause) "'Tell you one thing."

(IS) "What?"

(NO, extending hand,) "You've got a buddy for life!"

(IS, shakes his hand,) "Wow, thanks. That means a lot to me."

(NO) "Yeah, me too."

(Camera fades.)

(New scene: IS alone in his room, smiling, staring ahead, speaks to himself aloud in soliloquy,) "Wow! First the possibility of becoming a medical doctor, and then an awesome new buddy. Oh, boy! What next?"

(A knock on his door. IS responds,) "Yes?"

(Algebra teacher (AT) opens the door and peers through, speaking excitedly,)

"Zero Hero! A football win and an injury doesn't mean you can forget about -- ALGEBRA! Final exams and graduation coming up."

(IS, surprised, smiling,) "Oh, wow, come in! I've been thinking a lot about you." (Then embarrassed by his unplanned confession, tries to cover his words, speaks loudly,) "I mean, thinking of SCHOOL, ha, ha, and CLASS!"

(AT enters, dressed plainly in tee-shirt and below-the-knee skirt. She holds a textbook, paper tablet and pencil, initially smiling pleasantly, carefully closing the door behind her. But then turning and seeing his leg-cast, becomes worried, walks to IS, places her hand on his bare forearm, speaks with sympathy, "Oh, are you alright? I'm so sorry!"

(IS, surprised, looks at her hand, places his on top of it, then somewhat embarrassed, withdraws it quickly, answers,) "Thanks for your concern. I'm okay, just can't go anywhere for a few weeks." (He gazes about the room, continues,) "Sorry I can't offer you a chair – a bit crowded in here."

(AT, removing her hand from his arm,) "No problem. I'll just hop up here beside you. That way we both can use the lesson book."

(IS, speaking with the beginning of anxiety,) "Yes, Miss, whatever you say."

(AT perches on the bed beside and slightly behind him, one arm extended in support, the other holding the book; one leg stretched out beside his, the other dangling over the side of the bed, her skirt stretched tight across her thighs. The camera's view is their front, so both faces are in focus, but AT, behind IS, can't see his facial expressions in this sequence. As she settles into a comfortable position, her breast nudges against his back. She mumbles,) "Sorry." (She re-adjusts.

The camera shows him rather wide-eyed, looking over his shoulder,) "It's okay."

(AT then assumes a teaching tone, opening the text, pointing,) "Now remember, 'X' represents the unknown number, and your job is to find what it is." (Now speaking in a deep voice for emphasis,) "Your job is to uncover the unknown!" (Now speaking normally but with enthusiasm,) "That makes it kind of exciting, doesn't it?"

(While she has been discoursing, the camera focused in on IS's face, which progresses from uneasiness to overt anxiety. As he now speaks, slowly, grimacing, he stares down at her legs,) "My – job – is – to – uncover – the – unknown! Exciting!"

(AT, continuing instruction,) "So the first step is to form the equation, which as we said in class is like an old fashioned balance-scale, where they'd put some sugar on one side and weights on the other side, to see how much the sugar weighs." (Pause.)

(IS sighs heavily, stares back at her. AT, looking up at him, concerned,) "Are you okay? Something wrong?"

(IS, sighs again, speaking softly, anxious,) "Oh, boy, how do I say this? Miss, you see, I don't know anything about girls or women. I mean, Miss Hatfield was very strict with us. She said, 'Either you obey my rules or out you go.' She took good care of us and believe me, nobody wanted out. None of us had anywhere else to go. She gave a few innocent little parties, but I've never had anything like dates or stuff. I'm 'not schooled in the social graces.' That was a line I heard in a movie once." (He raises a finger for emphasis, speech softens, repeats,) " 'not schooled in the social graces.' But," (Speaks haltingly,) "you're so close to me, you smell so nice, we're all alone. I mean, I've always run away from where I might be alone with a pretty girl. But you can't run too far with a broken leg!" (Pause. He now brightens slightly, raises a finger again for emphasis, continues,) "Hey, I made that line up myself: 'Can't run too far with a broken leg.'" (Pause, again appears dejected, embarrassed,) "Sorry, Miss. You may have to help me. I don't quite know how to act."

(AT, now wide-eyed herself, sits forward, folds the book down, stares at him,) "Oh my heavens! A sensitive, honest boy!" (Pause, then reassuringly,) "It's okay. That's just normal. Just plain human feelings." (Pause. She studies him,) "How old are you?"

(IS) "Seventeen. No, wait! I almost forgot, with all the excitement. Today's my birthday! I'm eighteen years old." (Pause,) "And my birthday present is your coming to see me. Oh, I shouldn't have said that."

(AT) "Yes you should have. That's nice." (Pause,) "I love being your – eighteenth – eighteenth! birthday present." They stare at each other, he anxiously. Her frown gradually melts into a soft smile, the wide stare drifts to partly closed eyes, breathing deepens slightly.

(IS) "Sorry to be so much trouble."

(AT, now gently,) "You're not trouble. No trouble at all."

(She arises from the bed, lays the book aside, slowly walks over to the door, removes a "Do Not Disturb" sign from the inner-knob, opens the door, glances about, places the sign on the outer-knob, closes and locks the door and turns off the light. She walks back to the bed and once again sits beside

him, speaking softly, smiling,) "It's okay. Take my hand ."
(He takes it.

The camera has followed her during this sequence. It now slowly leaves them, panning gradually up the wall of the room behind the bed, the ambience moderately darkened with the lamp off, a single ray of sunlight entering through an unshaded window, reflecting off a mirror on the clothes-dresser and onto the ceiling. There a large fan revolves slowly, the light-ray through it casting a rotating shadow onto the ceiling. As the camera has panned up the wall, stopped and fixed at the revolving ceiling-shadow, the voice of IS is heard, initially softly,) "Oh, wow." (Pause, then excitedly,) "GOOD GRIEF!" (Pause, then again softly,) "Oh, my heavens."

(New scene: camera still focused on the revolving ceiling-fan shadows, but the shadow has shifted slightly, indicating a small passage of time. The sound track now reveals an audible quality to their breathing.)

(IS) "Miss! Your breath now has a funny, musky scent."

(AT, speaking slowly with a deepened, throaty quality.) "That happens."

(IS) "Miss! Your voice has changed."

(AT, breathing heavily,) "You can call me by my first name – Venus."

(New scene. Camera still fixed on the slowly revolving ceiling-shadow, but the shadow has now shifted considerably farther, indicating a larger time-passage. Silence. The camera shifts again down the wall to IS and AT in bed, propped up on pillows, discreetly covered by a sheet, smiling, regarding each other.)

(IS) "Are you okay?" (Rises slightly.)

(AT, closes eyes,) "I am a-one, okay, fine-fine, good-good-good."

(IS) "Wow, that's amazing! Is that what people do?"

(AT) "Some people, some times."

(IS) "Is it any different without a broken leg?"

(Pause. AT, answering,) "The principle is the same." (Both laugh.)

(IS, looking and speaking directly into the camera,) "Gee, sure a lot of things happen when you break your leg!"

(Camera fades, ending scene.)

(Transient secondary-title screen)

-- The Musician --

(Explanatory notation followed by resumption of action)

Three weeks later -- Central High School Graduation Night

(Camera fades to new scene. A married couple, CM and wife CW, age forties, are in their bedroom dressing for the graduation ceremony. CM implores CW,) "Why don't you go and I'll stay home? I'll even do the dishes!"

(CW, sitting at her dressing table, exasperated,) "Oh, stop it! You promised."

(CM, still complaining,) "But did you see this?" (Showing her the graduation program, continues,) "They have a student-violinist playing Paganini's 'Perpetual Motion'! This music was written in the early eighteen-hundreds, in Italy, one of the most difficult violin-concert pieces ever. No student could even attempt 'Perpetual Motion'. She couldn't play it at half-speed – probably could at quarter-speed, but then it would sound like a barn dance." (He looks pleadingly at his wife, who glares at him silently in return. He throws up his hands in surrender,) "Okay! Okay! I'll go!" (He then tightens a necktie about his neck, feigning distress,) "Gasp! Gasp! Choke! Choke!"

(CW resumes dressing,) "I refuse to look at your silliness."

(Camera fades to new scene. Student violinist (SV) in her wheelchair, the American Indian athlete (IA) and the student artist (AS) arrive at the graduation auditorium, well-dressed for the occasion.

(SV, to IA and AS,) "I have to admit, somewhat nervous playing in front of a crowd. But I have a plan to generate a little laugh first, which might lighten things a bit. I have an electronic tone-amplifier, which I use in tuning." (She shows the small box-like device,) "I will 'introduce' it initially, as if it were a person."

(IA) "That should generate some chuckles."

(SV) "I'll warn the ushers, maybe they can tell a few of the crowd to expect a comic moment."

(AS) "Sure, we can too."

(New scene, inside the auditorium packed with graduating seniors'

152

families and friends. On stage are the American Indian athlete (IA) and "number-one" athlete (NO) standing together, near the artist-student (AS). A master-of-ceremonies at podium with microphone addresses the crowd,) "Now in review, we have the two special athletic scholarships for college, awarded to our pair of spectacular performers," (motions IA and NO to step forward, "and then a full scholarship in fine art to that young painter who dropped in on us from Miss Hatfield's School like a bombshell!" (Motions to AS,) "Let's have a big hand for all three of them!" (Applause. After it subsides he continues,) "For a special treat, the next program-event is a musical number from another former student of Miss Hatfield –" (voice becomes muffled as camera pans backstage, focuses on SV in her wheelchair with violin, bow, and box-like tone amplifier on her lap. She wheels onto center-stage amid mild transient applause, sets the amplifier onto a small table, arranges music onto a music stand, picks up her violin.

Camera shifts from SV to CM and CW, now seated in the audience. CM, trying to avoid detection, is cautiously placing cotton in his ears. CW notices this and slaps his leg,) "Now stop that!"

(CM sighs, looks upward imploringly and removes the cotton. Camera again to SV as she prepares to play, placing a white handkerchief between her chin and the violin's chin-piece, a practice of some concert performers. CM, again looking upward, speaking softly, "Oh no! Not the handkerchief-under-the-chin bit. Oh, spare me, spare me!" (CW glares at him disapprovingly.

Camera to SV. She pushes a button on the amplifier-box; a clear tone is heard which she duplicates on the violin with a slight adjustment of several strings. She turns to the audience,) "This is my friend Tommy-the-Tone. He lives in this little box and helps me in tuning."

(The audience is silent. The laughter she had anticipated is not forthcoming. She sighs, and in preparation for her work, bows a short, very fast and complex flourish as her final portion of tuning and warm-up. The camera back to CM who is stunned by the flourish, sits forward, staring, speaks openly,) "Did you hear that? Did you see that?"

(The following is an intensely dramatic sequence which must be staged and directed skillfully, with a blend of complex audio, acting, and camera art. SV commences her performance to a quiet audience. Paganini's 'Perpetual Motion' is from the start extremely rapid and intricate, demanding almost unparalleled virtuosity by the performing artist.

Camera focuses firstly on SV's playing, then her face reflecting intense concentration, then shifting to close-up of the music sheets on a stand before her, with their complexity of musical notation. It then shifts to CM

153

in the audience; staring, engrossed, talking aloud to himself,) "No – she can't be doing this. It's impossible. Some kind of audio trick." (He slowly arises from his seat, inches toward the aisle, CW trying unsuccessfully to restrain him as he continues,) "There must be some kind of hidden recording." (He reaches the aisle, now the audience is murmuring, noticing him.

The camera picks up several of them speaking in soft tones,) "This must be the comic-part they warned us about."

"That guy some comedian we were told would happen?"

"Is this a funny interlude?" (Gradually, slight laughter is heard, and as CM continues toward the stage talking more loudly, the audience's interest in him and its laughter grows. The camera shifts back to close-up of the music sheet on the stand, indicating SV's concentration, she unaware of the growing background noise.

Suddenly the music sheets shake violently as the camera is focused in on them. The camera quickly backs off to show CM shaking SV's shoulder in disbelief; the appearance of sheet-music movement was actually SV's movement.

SV ceases playing, looks up, stunned at CM standing over her, looks out in horror at the audience now openly laughing as if on cue, mistaking this all for a comic act.

SV drops the violin and bow onto her lap, wheels herself quickly off to backstage, weeping bitterly in her assumed disgrace, leaving CM standing, staring after her, perplexed, the audience's laughter dwindling, also reflecting confusion. Camera shifts back to SV, now behind the curtain and out of the audience's view, crying hysterically. She is near to a steel post, part of the backstage structure. Camera now in slow-motion with sound muted, focuses on her as she picks the violin off of her lap, and grasping the thin neck of the instrument with both hands, swings it violently like a baseball bat, smashing it to pieces against the post. Still in slow motion, the camera backs off, showing the three senior students, IS (now in a lower-leg walking cast), AS and NO racing to her aid. Reaching her, they lift her bodily from the wheelchair, almost as in a dance, consoling and comforting; her arms go round them, she still crying, eyes closed, the mangled violin falling slowly to the floor. The three lower her gently back into her chair, she now more softly weeping, they gently caressing her in sympathy.

Camera, now back to full-motion and sound, shifts again to CM standing center-stage, wide-eyed in the realization of what has strangely transpired, the audience murmuring in confusion. He addresses them in a serious direct tone,) "Now to explain this bizarre incident, I begin by saying, some of you know me, I am First Violinist and Concert Master of our City

Symphony Orchestra, and the violin is a big part of my life. I humbly ask your forgiveness for this really gross interruption of tonight's program." (Pause) "To get us back on track, I would like each of you to do a simple thing. I want you all just to close your eyes, now." (Pause, silence, he closes his eyes, continues,) "Okay, now think back only a few moments ago, before I so rudely behaved. Think back, remember what was happening then." (Pause, total silence, camera in wide-angle view of CM and audience. Gradually applause begins, softly, then growing in volume, terminating in a standing ovation, eyes open, includes CM.

Camera shifts backstage to SV, wide-eyed at hearing the applause, dries her tears. The three seniors wheel her back to center-stage as ovation continues. CM holds up his hands as a signal; noise dwindles, audience seats. CM continues into the microphone, addresses SV,) "Now you can hear and see their true reaction to your playing! Their laughter had been at me! I was the clown!"

(Loud voice from his wife, CW, from the audience,) "You can say that again!"

(Audience laughs transiently, CM continues,) "My wife knows me only too well." (Now addressing SV,) "I have just one word to describe my reaction to your performance tonight. I am astounded!" (Pause) "So, tell us about yourself – what do you plan with the violin?"

(SV) "I know this sounds wild, but I have always hoped to become a concert performer. When she was young, Miss Hatfield was a promising classical violinist, and I have always hoped to take up where she left off. She gave me lessons daily, as far back as I can remember." (Pause,) "Sir, you said the violin is a big part of your life: I can tell you simply, the violin *is* my life."

(CM, smiling,) "Oh, I am so happy to hear that! And perhaps you'll even forgive me for my bad act."

(SV, also smiling,) "I do, Sir."

(CM, continuing,) "Well I can tell you this: from now on, you don't have to worry about a thing. I'll arrange it all: auditions, coaching, management – even a new violin. And my wife and I will work with you for other needs you may have."

(SV) "Thank you, Sir."

(CM) "Have you ever played in public before?"

(SV) "No."

(CM) "Well, I'm going to make a prediction: many years from now, toward the end of a long and spectacular stage career, you'll be interviewed by a reporter, who will ask, 'And do you remember the very first time you played before a public audience?" Then a distant look will come into your eyes, you'll pause a moment, and with a slight smile, you'll answer, 'Yes, actually I do recall. It was rather unusual."

(Audience laughter)

(CM) "Now, you didn't get to finish your piece. By chance, my own violin is in the trunk of our car. May I ask my good wife to please fetch it for us?"

(Camera cuts, pause, returns showing CW on stage, hands the violin case to CM. He carefully places it on a table, opens it and removes the instrument, offering it to SV. She stares at it, holds up her hands in a gesture of rejection, then,) "Oh my heavens! That's the most beautiful thing I've ever seen in my life. I'd be afraid to touch it, let alone play it."

(CM) "Well, you're right, it's not a Stradivarius, though close behind. But, okay to play it; here, I'll tune it for you." (He looks at the electronic amplifier-box, continues,) "This little guy was supposed to be the comic act, but instead, I was!" (Audience chuckles. CM activates the amplifier and tunes the violin, making minor adjustments on the string-knobs. He then hands her the violin rather ceremoniously. She cautiously accepts it, studying it, begins its placement. He hands her the bow, adding,) "Here is your own bow. Do you need to warm up?"

(SV) "No, I'm already pretty warm."

(Audience laughter. CM continues,) "Don't forget the handker-chief-under-the-chin. Yours is rather damp. Here's a clean one." (Offers her a handkerchief; she accepts and positions it. CM continues arranging the sheet music and positioning the stand,) "From the beginning, please."

(SV positions herself, smiles, gazes out over the audience, serenely confident of mastering the Paganini patiently awaiting her. At once and for the first time, she becomes totally aware of her life's destiny as a concert performer. Then her face reflects a quick mode-shift from relaxation to intense concentration as she begins to play. The music, furious and fast, dominates the scene over a hushed audience, the camera gently backing away from her face and slowly circling her. Her playing uniquely blends the written, timeless artistry with her own individual interpretive overlay, creating a stunningly beautiful effect onto the senses.

"Perpetual Motion" is a relatively short piece and at its conclusion the audience, awed by her brilliance and virtuosity, sits silent, transfixed, staring, unmoving. SV gives the violin and bow over to CM; her hands now folded, she totally tranquil, a Mona Lisa smile. Then the audience, awakening to reality, explodes into a thunderous standing ovation with shouts and whistles, SV now openly weeping tears of joy, acknowledging the audience and CM, bowing from the waist, blowing kisses, the camera slowly pulling back. A nicely-dressed young girl brings a colorful bouquet of flowers on-stage and presents it to the musician. She receives the flowers graciously and extracting several, hands one each to CM, AS, IS, and NO, they bowing appreciatively in acceptance. As applause continues, the camera focuses into the audience to the two teachers originally present in Prolog: TO and TT.)

(TT to TO,) "You remember awhile back we agreed that these Hatfield students were about to change 'old Central High' forever?"

(TO) "I'd say we were right on!" (They slap hands above heads in a "high-five" salute.) Camera pulls back from audience, which is still cheering. Noise slowly mutes and is replaced by the discordant high school marching-band music heard first in the opening scenes, as credits supervene.

The End

(Title screen followed by action)

– Letters // A Sequel // "X" –

(New scene: split-screen horizontally, the top portion silently show-ing action as described in the lower part, which is a series of hand-written letters between the student-athlete (SA), now in college, and his former algebra teacher (AT). The audios are "voice-overs," first a neutral com-mentator followed by her voice and then his, as they compose their notes sequentially. These personal letters scroll by below. When no action is writ-ten, the upper-screen shows the thoughtful writer, pen in hand.)

"He was surprised and rather upset, even a bit fearful, at receiving the first letter, having tried, unsuccessfully, to forget her. He initially stared at the envelope, but after opening and reading it, his frown softened into a slight smile."

"Rain, Greetings from Central High! I thought you might be interest-ed in some of the happenings at your Alma Mater. Opening football game was a tough loss to North High, 7-6. CHS kicked two field goals early, but in the waning seconds NHS threw a tremendous long pass and pulled it out. The radio-announcer still talks about your spring performance, 'That anonymous Zero-Hero!' Your former running coach is now assistant at the school. He has discarded his cane though still walks with a limp. The students love both – they are such foils! The head-coach is emotional and wildly demonstrative, his helper droll and factual. Even though the team lost, the students put on a giant rally for them.

Stay well, Venus"

"Venus, Thanks for the note – sounds like ol' Central High is as wooly and wild as ever! Pretty busy now with football starting plus studies, but here's a little happening you might find funny: yesterday I went to the head coach's office, knocked, entered and stated, 'Sir, I'd like to talk to you about baseball.'

He stared at the ceiling, sighed, then, 'If you weren't one of my prom-ising freshman players, I'd send you out of here with a kick in the pants! Our first FOOTBALL game only weeks away and – BASEBALL?'

'Sir, baseball in relation to football.'

'Alright, you've got thirty seconds.'

'Okay, in baseball they don't have a separate team of batters, the of-fense, and fielders, the defense. The same guys play both.'

'You've got twenty more seconds.'

'Sir, also remember way back in the early years of football, they wore leather helmets with no face masks.'

'Yeah, those players were tough!'

'Well, those same guys played both offense and defense, just like in baseball.'

'So?'

'Sir, I'm asking your permission for me to play offense AND defense now in football.'

Well, he stared at me, then got up and walked around the room mumbling to himself and gesturing with his hands, reminded me of my Central High head coach, wildly demonstrative. Then finally he put his face right in front of mine and shouted, 'Listen to me! You're not playing on any special teams – no kicking or receiving! Y' understand that?'

'Yessir!'

'And, d' ya know what the sportswriters will say about this? They'll fry me!'

'Yessir!'

'D' you realize you'll get twice the bruises and hits as any other player? AND you'll have to know BOTH game plans!'

'Yessir!'

Then he paused, backed off and spoke slowly, eyes half-closed, 'First play from scrimmage, defense, you're playing linebacker. First offense, tight end.'

'Yessir!"

'NOW GET OUT OF HERE!'

'Yessir!'

As I left he shouted, 'And don't ask permission to sell peanuts in the stands at half time, either!'

'Yessir!'

'And stop saying 'Yessir'!'

'Yessir! – I mean, okay!' And he threw a blackboard eraser at me as I went out the door.

Best, Rain"

"Their letters were short, sporadic and infrequent – sometimes months apart. They were 'chatty' and 'newsy' only, nothing even remotely romantic or emotional.

But they continued."

"Rain, I forgot to warn you, there at the "center of higher learning" (!!); watch out for those aggressive college girls. They like handsome athletes!

Cheers, Venus"

"Venus, Ha, ha, you mentioned "college girls"; I had a dinner-movie date with one last week. I almost fell asleep at the table, and then did in the dark theater! When I awakened, the movie was over and she had gone home. Surely I made a great impression on her!

Regards, Rain"

"Then, that next spring, a subtle change took place in their greetings; she noticed this, he didn't."

"Dear Venus, Now it's baseball time, and I find third-base perfect for me. The "hot corner"! Some of everything in that position. Looks like I'll be starting even though a freshman. Work-out hard, study hard, but I like it.

Be careful, Rain"

"Dear Rain, Congrats on baseball-starting! And good grades, too. I know 'The U' got their money's worth with your scholarship.

I'm proud of you, Venus"

"Dear V, Thanks for the kind words. I have no family, so you're my only cheerleader. And here's a little sports-irony: you may know that my school-team is known as "The Indians." No one here is aware that my father was a real Native-American 'Indian', Hopi Tribe. (I don't know about my mother — I was an orphan. I'll tell you about it sometime.)

I'm proud of my heritage! R."

"She read and re-read his letter, finding some solace in his words, though not sure why. Maybe it was his revealing to her something close, personal."

"Dear R, While you're doing such wonderful things, I also hear good news from other CHS grad-classmates. I read where your former football adversary-now-best-friend, Ty Shane, is really turning heads at the US Olympic Track Training Camp. Those fellow "Hatfield School" chums too – Maria D'Maya Sanchez received rave reviews for her European violin debut at London's Covent Garden. The critics really went wild over the same

Paganini she played at your graduation! And painter J'Jeune Altis won first prize at the Spring Abstract Competition for young artists in Berlin.
Stay well, V."

"Innocent and mild as these letters were, over time they had the result of   drawing the two ever-so-slightly closer; she realized this, he didn't.
Also it turned out they had many shared interests."

"Hi, Rain, time for only a quick note and greetings (along with a cup of coffee) from the Faculty Lounge before class. Just got in from swimming laps, hair still wet. My exercise most mornings.
Best, V."

"Dear V., Nice that you swim AMs. I've always embraced the ancient Greek credo, "Knowledge, Strength, Beauty."
'Bye, R."

"As he wrote these words, he suddenly caught himself thinking, `Venus has all three and then a whole lot more.`   But each time he thought of her, which was often, he would become somewhat confused and sometimes even a little depressed. He had grown up without a mother, though Miss Hatfield had provided for him nicely. Venus was older, and presumably wiser, and she did encourage him in school. Yet they had been lovers once."

"Dear R., Just in from dance-class, still in slippers! Did I tell you I teach classical ballet after school? One of my favorite activities. And get this – your former running-coach (now assistant in football) has talked me into a dance-class for the team. He said if I ever see you (!) to tell you and you'd understand.
Care, V."

"Hey, V! Wonderful that you teach ballet! You may be surprised to hear that I was assistant dance-instructor awhile back, when I worked part-time at the Rehab Hospital. We had a teacher for the patients and I helped. And I do understand the benefit of dance-class for athletes. Timing, coordination, etc. etc.
Stay good, R."

"Hi R. Whew! Just got in from rehearsals – worn out! Feet up! I'm coaching the seniors in their play "Romeo and Juliet." The boys love the fighting, the girls the romance. Fun + work.

All, V."

"Dear V. Sharespeare! Oh, wow! Good for you.

I've always preferred the classics. Timeless, not to mention educational and entertaining too. No doubt I'm the only player on our team who reads Shakespeare for pleasure.

Cheers, R."

"Then for awhile their missives took on a playful tone, a sure sign that more of – something – was developing between them."

"Dear R. I meant to ask, have you figured out what that strange, elusive-yet-compelling (even enticing!) "thing," "X," is by now?

Stay, V. (Your Algebra teacher!)"

"No, Venus/Teacher!! Advanced math + calculus are truly interesting, but I still haven't gleaned what that mystery-of-life, "X" is! I'll let you know when I've found out!

(?"Stay"? Is that supposed to be like in dog-training school? Here's a better one . I heard a German say it once:)

Addy-Ose, R."

"R., I do believe you mean the Spanish goodbye:

Adios, V.

PS 'Stay' means 'Stay the wonderful person you are.'"

"Dear V., OK! I stand corrected. But I met this Russian once, and when he left, he said, "Chow." I thought he was off to eat dinner.

Here's one I think is French:

Alf Weeder Sain, R."

"R. Oh, you slay me! "Ciao" is a vague European colloquial "goodbye," and "Auf Wiedersehen" is German for "'til we meet again."

I do believe foreign languages are not your forté.

Ciao, V."

"V. – So what does forté mean? Is it French for = 39 + 1? Here's one I know is spelled correctly; I read it in a book!
Bon voyage, R."

"R!! – 'Bon Voyage' is French for "Have a pleasant journey. And "for-té" is French, meaning "strength", from the Latin root "fort", as in an Army "fort."
How about NO closing, like,
V."

"VVVVVVVVVVVVV! NO closing is like a sundae without whipped-cream or a dance without music – NEIN! Here's one I think is Swedish :
Sayonara Senorita, Rain"

"Dear R, Oh, You have me confused -- now you're mixing Japanese (`goodbye`) and Spanish (`Miss`). How about something more conven-tional/American, like,
Fondly, Venus"

He ignored her request and simplified his closings.
Though the letters continued infrequently during his years at college, they never mentioned a wish or plan to meet again.
Except once:

"Dear V., Only a short note, just in from late study. I like to cook, but this little hot-plate and mini-fridge in my tiny apartment don't permit much. Thank heaven for canned food!
Always, R"

"Dear R, I worry you're not getting enough to eat. I love to cook also and if I could ever see you again, I'd prepare you a nice meal.
'Bye, V"

"He didn't reply for a protracted interval and never answered her in-vitation.
She realized her mistake and didn't repeat it.
But he did write again, later."

"Dear V, Haven't "talked" to you in awhile – hope you are well. I'm battered, playing both offense and defense, but we did make it to a bowl invitation. This will be my last football game, able to graduate in three years, right after baseball season.

Cheers, R."

"Dear R, So proud of you, "Most Valuable Player" in the bowl game! And history being made, as you were on the losing team (by one measly point!) But an obvious choice, as you were the only outstanding player on the field, all the others just 'good' or 'fair'.

Wow! V."

"Hi, V., Time flys! Now my final baseball season is going well. Looks like we'll make it to the College World Series.

Study, baseballs, books, bats, etc. etc.

Sleepy now, R."

"Rain! Rain! Good grief! That College World Series -- what a dramatic exit from your school athletics! I watched it all on TV and cheered myself hoarse.

I want to write this all down so I don't forget the details. (I save all your letters and copies of mine.) Here goes:

Your team has won its way up the ladder to the top two teams, in a final two-out-o three games to determine the series winner. Each team has won one game, so now it's the final, deciding contest for the championship! It's been a "pitchers' duel" so far, with you ahead 1 - 0 (by virtue of your home run). But, it's the last of the ninth inning, AND they have bases loaded, no outs with their 'power-hitter' at bat! Their coach must have thought he could get it over quickly in such a good situation and secretly signaled a hit-and-run play. Then a scorching line-drive just inside the base-line, you make a spectacular diving catch, step on the bag, tag out the incoming base-runner and trot off the field! A historic, winning, unassisted triple play at third base! It even took a moment for the officials to realize what had happened. Then there's that silly opposing-player racing around second, not knowing that, in a flash, the play was over, the inning was over, the game was over and the College World Series was over!

Oh, Rain, If I had been there in the stands, I'd have vaulted the fence, fought through the mob and kissed you!

You are indeed amazing!!

Love, V"

(As this baseball play-action is described in her letter, the upper-portion of the screen shows it happening, silently, in slow-motion for that short sequence.)

"He cringed reading her letter, particularly the last line and closing, again confused and a little depressed over his conflicted feelings for her. But after reflecting somberly about his life and future, he sighed, sat down and forced himself to compose what would be his last letter to her."

"Dear Venus, You're right – that was a wild finale to my college sports, though I plan always to work-out and keep a good 'bod'. Some really attractive offers from the pro's, both football and baseball, hard to turn down. I even got a nice invitation to join the professional dance company I worked with Saturdays at the Rehab Hospital. They wanted me to start a new program offering dance instruction to high-school athletic teams around the state. An interesting idea! But I'm committed to becoming a doctor and don't want to get sidetracked.

Venus, I sincerely want to thank you again for everything – your interest in me and encouragement (even cheering!), and our friendly banter that always brought a smile. These have been three tough years and your letters have surely helped tremendously to keep me on track.

But now I'm starting a new life-chapter.

I'll never forget you, Venus – never.

I wish you the very best.

Stay well, Venus, ever – ever.

Rain"

"She cried, reading, and re-reading, his emotional words; almost as if they meant a final farewell.

Almost…

But not quite…

Then she made her decision."

Transient title screen:

College Graduation Day

New scene: Outdoor graduation ceremony, bright sunlight, graduates in black academic caps and gowns seated in front rows, guests behind. The Dean stands at podium before a microphone, "And so on this highly significant day, in conclusion, I'm reminded of a cartoon I once saw: the graduates are in line to receive diplomas, and one of them says to another, 'There are still one or two things I'm not entirely clear on." (Audience laughter.) "So I hope each of you has a lifetime of learning ahead. I want to thank friends and families for attending today, and again congratulations and best wishes to you new graduates for passing this difficult and momentous life-milestone. My final-final word to you is, remember this: there's a big exciting world out there, filled with joy as well as sadness, both laughter and tears. My advice is: don't sit back and miss it all. Get out there – AND – JUST – DO IT!"

(Loud standing ovation, graduates shaking hands and hugging each other, some in tears.) Camera focuses in on Rain, mingling transiently with colleagues, finally walking silently away from the crowd, holding his diploma. The camera closes in on his face, relaxed with slight smile. Then the loud voice of Venus behind him, "Rain! Rain!" A close-up of his face, obvious instant voice recognition. He grimaces. Fear. Wide-eyed; he stops in his tracks. He turns, faces her; she runs toward him, she well-dressed for the occasion, smiling, arms outstretched, "Oh, Rain! I just had to come and see you graduate! I'm so proud of you, in only three years! And highest honors, both scholastic and athletic!"

He backs away, arms at his sides, anxious, fearful, "Venus!"

She stops, her smile fades, arms drop, slight frown, "What's wrong? Am I interrupting something?"

"No, not interrupting, " He is startled, staring.

"But isn't this a happy occasion?" (Puzzled)

"Yes, happy, graduation -- " (Pause, he tries to calm his emotions, forces a slight smile,) "You look nice."

"Thanks." (Pause, staring at each other, he fearful, she now anxious also. She continues,) "Let's both sit over here." (Motions toward a bench. They sit; he edges away from her. She,) "What?"

(He turns his head away, closes eyes, speaking emotionally,) "Oh, boy. How do I say this?"

(She, now a slight smile,) "You used those same words on me once before."

(He, haltingly,) "I know I was just a little boy, desperately in love with his teacher, older and unreachable, but I can't help it. I can't forget you, even though it's been three years." (Eyes now moist,) "And seeing you now brings it all back even stronger. Starting med-school here soon, four hard years, financially too, and even the years to follow, on into orthopedic surgery. Oh, boy."

(Longer pause, then she, speaking distinctly,) "A high school near here has an opening for an algebra teacher." (Pause; he remains secluded.) "Did you hear what I just said?"

"No."

"I said," (Repeats. He looks up, studies her, confused. She continues, "Rain, listen to me! I can't forget you either. That's why I wrote you, researched out that job, came here now. I've had boyfriends through the years but you touched me in some strange magical way." (Pause) "Rain, for heaven's sake, I'm only five years older than you! What difference does it make? I'm not 'unreachable'! I know times ahead will be hard, but I can help. That new job pays really well." (Pause, her eyes now moist also,) "Rain, I want to be with you." (Rain is now staring at her, slapping his own cheek and blinking his eyes rapidly. She, lightening slightly,) "You did that once before, in class." (He stops after a few moments. Pause. They sit immobile, staring at each other. Then she,) "Three years ago you quoted lines to me from a movie – remember?"

"I remember every word, every detail."

"Well, now I have a movie-line for you. An old black-and-white film, great actress, maybe Marlene Dietrich. The couple is sitting there staring at each other in total silence. Finally she says, "Kiss me, you fool!"

(He leaps forward, takes her head in both hands, kisses her repeatedly, she holding him also. He, amazed at this life-altering surprise, pulls away slightly, stares wide-eyed, deeply at her,) "Jesus!"

She, staring wide-eyed also, "No, Venus!"

He, now a soft smile, at once resolving his convoluted feelings for her, chuckles, "Oh, I've regarded you in such awe! It's wonderful to laugh with you now!"

"Don't laugh too long; I liked what you were doing before."

"But I have to tell you why I was slapping my own face back there in your class."

"What?"

"I imagined you lecturing at the blackboard wearing only a bra and panties!"

"Oh, that's so funny! But you don't have to just imagine me ever again. I'm here to stay."

They embrace again, but then once more he pulls back momentarily, "Algebra is a wonderful part of life!"

"Indeed!"

"It's taken me three years, but I do believe I've finally learned what that elusive thing 'X' is." (Mixed laughter and embracing; camera fades to new scene with transient explanatory title screen.)

Twenty-Five Years Later

New scene: a large bare stage, curtains drawn to the side, the backdrop mural suggests a small Spanish village with hill-tops distantly. A full audience is silent, awaiting the performance. Sub-title appears transiently below: "FANDANGO, Music by Antonio Soler (1729-83, Spanish), Choreography by Marius Petipa (1818-1910, French-Russian)."

The orchestral music then begins: this is a fiery folk-dance in three-quarter time, with continuous rapid tempo throughout. The performers appear from opposite sides of the stage: a young couple, both in colorful Spanish peasant garb; he with tambourine and head scarf, she with short skirt, point-shoes and bright accoutrements. The two, widely smiling, emanate happiness as they dance in classical rapid ballet format, alternating solos and pas-de-deux over a fifteen-minute sequence, culminating in his assisting her in a leaping turn ("grand jeté en tournant"), then a classic final pose together, he on bended knee, she outstretched and balanced on his upper leg. Thunderous applause as they now stand, bow, and make humble gestures of gratitude to the audience. A young girl approaches them from the wings and hands her a multicolored floral bouquet. She picks and presents her partner a flower as applause continues. An announcer with microphone approaches the two; clapping subsides.

"So there you have it ladies and gentlemen, patrons of the arts: our winners in this year's international competition for young dancers in classical ballet." (Applause returns, finally closing. He addresses the two,) "Congratulations to you both. I can foresee a wonderful future for each of you in the world of professional dance. And now they wish to add a few words." (He hands the microphone over to her.)

"Thank you, thank you, gracious audience, and we appreciate our wonderful teachers through the years, and the sponsors of this event."

(Transient applause. She hands the microphone to her partner.)

(He speaks emotionally,) "But most of all, we want to thank our mother and father, for, for EVERYTHING! Dr. and Mrs. Rain Meadow, please stand!" (Points to front-row, center. Applause re-erupts, including the two dancers. Camera focuses in on the parents as they stand and face the audience, holding hands, raising them as a form of salute. They are older now, slightly grey, but still a handsome pair. They turn and face their daughter and son, then to each other and kiss. The camera focuses in on them in close-up and freezes as the sound of applause dwindles and is replaced by background high-school marching band music, similar to that earlier in the play, as credits supervene.)

The End

"Sorry, I Didn't Mean To Stare -- "

short story

She was thirty-six years old, he was twenty-eight. They stood alone in opposite corners of the old elevator, ascending slowly. Studying her "to-do" list, she felt a vague sense of unease. Looking up, his eyes were transfixed on hers. He quickly averted them, closed them, dropping his head slightly, touching the bridge of his nose, "Sorry, I didn't mean to stare."

"What were you staring at?" -- glad to be distracted from her list.

Glancing at his wristwatch, "Oh, only seven-thirty, and already I'm in trouble."

"You're not in trouble!" Slightly amused.

Looking at her again, still a serious tone, "You reminded me of someone I knew long, long ago."

He crossed over and read her name tag, "RN, Director Neuro-Intensive Care." As she read his also, he continued, "I'm a new extra-duty general surgery resident, which means filling in the gaps as needed in the operating room, while I try to get into a cardiac-surgery specialty training fellowship." He stared at her again, and for the first time, a slight smile, "I'll bet when you were little, they called you 'carrot-top.'"

"They still do!"

A slight pause, then, "Do you always wear bangs?"

"Do you like them?"

"I love them."

(On rare occasion, two who meet by chance will feel an intense attraction for each other, strong enough to surprise or even frighten them. The consequence may be comic, happy, sad, tragic, all -- or nothing.)

The aged elevator jerked to a stop, the door creaked open and a hospital-bed rolled in, with patient aboard and nurses attending. Intravenous fluids were flowing; a cardiac monitor lay beside him on the bed. He was being ventilated en-route, a nurse periodically squeezing the plastic bag to his endotracheal tube. Slow to recover postoperatively, he had finally progressed sufficiently for transfer to a second-level care ward.

Eyeing the two elevator occupants, the team leader announced loudly, "Sorry folks, the new hospital promises bigger and faster elevators, but in the meantime this is a game called (singsong), 'Get-to-know-your-fellow-citizens-more-closely,' and we'll all squee-eeze in here!"

By necessity he was pressed up against her in the corner, his face slightly above hers. She flushed, feeling his nearness and warmth. He studied the bright red hair falling over her forehead and the soft wrinkles about her pale green eyes. Locked together while the old elevator creaked and swayed rhythmically as it rose, they were as lovers dancing to a slow waltz.

Then the cell-phone rang in the pocket of his short white doctor's coat, worn over surgical scrub clothes. She too wore a white jacket, oversized and loose-fitting, over a more formal, neat, management-level dress. Years before, she had learned to wear extra-large clothes, hiding her female form to prevent stares from the males of all stations in life who seemed to parade endlessly in droves through the hospital halls; stares she had endured in school as an adolescent.

As he brought the phone up between them, he realized her ruse.

"Sorry," he mumbled.

"It's okay," a light gasp as sensations ricocheted throughout her body.

He had developed a keen sense of smell from years in hospitals and clinics, with their varieties of odors and essences.

He thought he detected a slight aura of passion on her breath.

"Right on!" He spoke loudly into the phone, "Your friendly resident is on the way."

The elevator stumbled to a stop; the patient with nurse-entourage departed.

He stepped out, and after quickly glancing about to ensure privacy, blew her a kiss.

Her heart raced.

That afternoon she walked across the bridge corridor to the clinic building, towing a two-wheeled cart of patient records, her slightly bowed legs taking long strides. She reflected back to her strange sudden attraction for the young doctor in the elevator that morning. But she also, for the first time, sensed a vague fear – formless but present, as one might perceive the almost-visible outline of a ship in dense fog.

He came quickly from behind her, touching her arm. She knew it was he even before seeing him, and again her heart pounded and she flushed. No Greeting; instead his asking simply, "What time do you get off work?"

"Oh, six – "

"Do you know the 'Half-Moon Bar' up the street at Five Points?"

"I've seen it."

"Meet me there at six-thirty." In contrast to her, he walked in quick short steps. Speeding on ahead, waving over his shoulder while not looking

171

back, "Don't be late."

"But wait, wait – "

He did not slow to listen.

That evening they arrived almost simultaneously. Her face reflected anxiety. She laid her hand on his arm, "I can't now, no -- "

He paused, then, "Oh, Madam, I must admit I was stunned by your beauty at first seeing you, then tricked you into coming here, hopefully to know you better. But now I see in your eyes I have only brought you unhappiness. I apologize. Therefore I shall exit your life at this time." (During important discourse he had a way of speaking rapidly and formally in high-pitched tones, utilizing technical terms; a habit carried over from the operating room.)

He turned to go.

"No, please, don't – just later," her eyes now hopeful.

He arrived at her apartment promptly. Thirty minutes later they were in her bed, tearing at each other, grasping, guttural sounds, as if this primordial act could wash away the unhappy lives, the injuries, the pains that swirled about them episodically in the hospital. Errors, misunderstandings, deaths.

Then his cell-phone rang – a most inopportune time.

"Hey, Pal, I know you're off-call, but hear this! A twelve-year old kid is riding one of those motorized-tricycle jobs in the woods, too fast I'm sure, hits a rock, thrown out, lands on a stump about a centimeter across. There he is lying impaled on a stick through his chest! His buddy calls nine-eleven and luckily the EMTs sawed off the stump instead of trying to pull it out. Can you imagine, the kid is lying here on a stretcher with a stake through his heart! He looks like Dracula! He's actually awake with a blood pressure. The echocardiogram shows it's through the atria, but missed the valves and major coronaries and has sealed things off. Surprisingly he's conversant and taking it well, though the parents have freaked out and are with the chaplain. So we've got a real chance for a cure. Plan to put him on peripheral by-pass, go straight in anteriorly, tie off everything sequentially, a cardiac purse-string suture around the stake and then slow careful extraction while keeping the purse-string tight. Now the 'Big Man' knows how much you like weird-o cases, so he's invited you to scrub-in as second assist. But you'll have to hurry, the blood-bank almost has a match."

Because of his evening schedule: one night first-call, next night second-, third night off, they spent each third night alone together.

Except once.

"I can't," he phoned, "sad death. Thirteen-year-old girl, terminal inoperable heart disease. She was alone, no family, perfectly lucid, the chaplain and nurse were with us. She knew she was dying, said she wasn't afraid and thanked us for trying to help, asked that her ashes be scattered over the children's playground at City Park, place of her happiest memories. She was staring at my face when the monitor straight-lined, her eyes glazed and she was gone. Normally I handle this type thing, but this one got to me. I just have to be alone awhile, in the dark."

"Oh, I'm so sorry – I know, I know. I've been down that road so many times myself. But just remember, she wasn't alone; you were with her."

Together they avoided talk of the past or future or of controversial subjects. Instead they dwelt on hospital matters and patient cases. Not realizing it on a conscious level, they avoided conversing about topics which might uncover disagreements and so jeopardizing their happiness together.

They spent a lot of time in her bed, not talking at all.

Several weeks later he arrived at her apartment early and was greeted by her two teen-age daughters, back from a visit with their father.

"Oh, I can't believe it! Three beautiful red-headed gals living in the same house!

The girls beamed.

He entered. "I'm a doctor. What do you guys do?"

"Oh, nothing, you know, like go to school and some other stuff. I'm the athlete-type and she's the smart one," answered the older girl.

"Great! The perfect combination! Now 'smarty' teaches 'sporty' how to study better and 'sporty' teaches 'smarty' how to get physical! Then each has the two most important features of a mature person, a sharp mind and a great bod."

"You're forgetting the third element, which may be the most important – the soul, or feeling, or heart, whatever you wish to call it. Otherwise we are only muscular computers," replied the younger girl.

"Good grief! You are smart. A teen-age philosopher!"

Later after the girls' mother arrived, they all sat down to dinner.

A square wooden table with four chairs.

A simple meal in a small modestly-appointed room.

Silence.

The two girls stared at each other across the table, the lovers the same. Slight smiles.

The girls had the feeling something wonderful was happening, but not knowing what it might be.

Acting spontaneously and intuitively, he arose from the table, went to the younger girl, bent over, took both her hands into his and kissed them, then to the older girl the same, and to their mother. He kissed her on the lips – a light kiss but long. He sat down again and for the first time in his life felt reverent and wondered if they blessed their meals.

Then his cell-phone rang.

"Sorry to bother you, Doctor, but this is overseas-incoming and he insisted I 'ring you up' as he put it. Go ahead, Sir. He's on the line."

"Good morning, Doctor, or for you, good evening. This is the Chief Registrar at London Central Hospital. As you know, we have on file here your application for our two-year cardiac surgical training program. We've had an unexpected opening and would like you to come join us. The only problem is we need you to travel on over as soon as possible. With holidays coming up, there's a lengthy queue of elective surgeries on school children with congenital defects. This will be a sterling learning experience for you and prepare you to be a fully-trained independent heart surgeon."

She cried bitterly and long, for she was deeply wounded.
She *knew*.
Her daughters consoled her.

The next morning, riding the elevator up to her office, she read her "To Do" list:

1. New admission: twelve-year old male quadriplegic from shallow-pool diving injury.

2. Meet lawyers re: liability suit: parents claim inadequate care in death of self-induced drug-overdose admission.

3. Conference: doctors' group complaining of insufficient nursing staff.

4. Meet pharmacists re: outdated computer system for medication management.

None of the parties involved had the slightest awareness that they were enabling her to maintain a functional level of emotional stability throughout the day.

He, now in a different world, was swept up in the unrelenting maelstrom of science and human drama which enshrouds a doctor learning the specialty of cardiac surgery.

Weeks later, however, he was reminded of her while walking by the Burn Unit of the hospital's Pediatric Wing. Glancing through an interior window, he happened to observe a nurse applying soothing cream to the badly burned skin of an infant: the intensity of her expression and the deliberate, smooth, studied movement of the nurses' hands onto the child were as a symphony conductor working through a slow difficult passage; they reflected a degree of tenderness and compassion uncommon even on the Pediatric Ward.

Those hands reminded him of her caresses.

But reality blew away his reverie and urged him on to see his own patient, an infant born with a simple heart defect preventing complete blood oxygenation, rendering the child bluish-colored with stunted growth. But now it was old enough for total correction and the strong probability of future normality.

He hurried on for the pre-operative evaluation.

They never saw each other or communicated with one another again.

Years later, while riding the elevator up to her office one morning, she caught herself looking over the top of her "To Do" list, staring at a young doctor talking on a cell-phone.

Her eyes misted over as she recalled.

Intersection // Multidimensional

– A Classic Tale, Dark…

Screenplay

Muses present for the creation of this script:
- American playwright Tennessee Williams
- Swedish film-writer/director Ingmar Bergman
- Viennese psychoanalyst Sigmund Freud
- Christian Apostle Saint John
- Ancient Greek poet Sophocles

(Opening Inscription)

"Heaven from all creatures hides
    The Book of Fate,
All but the page prescrib'd
    Their present state."
            — Alexander Pope (English poet, 1688-1744)

Dramatis Personae

(Major)

– Rex, age twenty-two years, dressed in blue jeans and tee shirt, gold-colored but faded. He wears a billed-cap with the headband containing a barely visible vertical-stripe pattern.

– Jo, age forty-two, wearing a simple off-white, below-knee dress. The belt sags somewhat in front, and the lower-body portion over the hips is noticeably darker in color. She wears a brown headband, patterned; hair straight and shoulder-length, light brown. No makeup; bare-legged with simple sandals, her feet noticeably muddy. She carries only a small paper sack.

(Minor)

– Gasoline-station attendant.

– Bus-ticket clerk

– "Death", in black total-body costume, with skull and bones painted white.

– Third grade class of Sioux Indian children.

– First-year medical-school human anatomy laboratory class of sixty or so students with instructor.

[Black and white filming to emphasize the story-line without distraction; no background music. Subtitles throughout, as some lines are whispered and barely audible.]

Opening scene: Small town in the mountains of western Montana, a combination of tiny gasoline station and bus-stop. Time is contemporary, early autumn, late afternoon. An attendant is fueling Rex's medium-sized recreational vehicle (RV), which has a flat snub-nosed front with tall wind-shields similar to those of a modern city bus.

Rex: (To attendant,) "Yeah, been out camping awhile, my last taste of freedom. Like getting married in two weeks."

Attendant: "Really. Who's the girl?"

Rex: "Well, actually it's not a girl."

Attendant: "Hey, you don't mean you're one of those – "

Rex: (Laughing.) "No, No! I'm starting med-school, and I know that's a big-time commitment. The medical profession is a very jealous spouse –" (Interrupted by Jo.)

Jo: (Standing outside at the bus-ticket window, near Rex and the attendant. She speaks to the ticket clerk inside the window, speaking softly, distraught,) "Thirty dollars for a one-way ticket to Styx County? I only have twenty dollars. "

Clerk: "Sorry, Ma'am. Rates have gone up."

Jo: (Turns away, sobbing lightly, unsteady; to herself, barely audible,) "What can I do?"

Rex: "Wait, Ma'am. I'm heading that way, across Styx, maybe I can give you a lift."

Jo: (Recovering slightly; regards him,) "That would be nice."

Rex: "Are you alone?"

Jo: "Yes." (Pause.) "Yes, I'm alone, ha, ha, yes, – alone." (She laughs a soft ironic laugh, which degenerates into a barely visible type of silent weeping, which then progresses to a detached, withdrawn persona; looking away blankly. This type of response from her will be repeated episodically throughout the play.)

Rex: (Speaking to Jo while paying the attendant. Preoccupied, he has not noticed her emotional distress,) "Well, okay then, get your things and climb aboard."

Jo: "I don't have any things." (Pause, then distantly,) "I gave every-thing away." (Another pause, then looking at her feet,) "Oh dear, I must have walked through some mud. My feet and sandals are dirty. I don't want to soil your nice RV."

Rex: (Picking up and turning on a nearby garden-type hose,) "No problem. I was just topping off the radiator, so hop up onto the seat and dangle your feet over, and I'll rinse them off for you."

Jo: (Doing so, removing her sandals. Speaking softly,) "Thank you."

Rex: (He finishes rinsing, turns off the water and replaces the hose as she swings her legs into the cab and closes her door. He climbs into the driver's seat, closes the door and, smiling, extends his hand,) "I'm Rex."

Jo: (Furrows her brow, studies him intently. Pause,) "That was my son's name." (Recovering slightly, she shakes his hand,) "Mine's Jo."

Rex: (Now, for the first time regarding her more seriously,) "That is a coincidence! My mother's name was Jo." (She returns his look briefly, then stares blankly out of the side window as he starts the engine and eases the RV onto the road. They begin an almost continuous climb in largely deserted mountainous terrain. A somewhat awkward silence, then an attempt at conversation,) "Have family in Styx County?" (Jo remains silent, staring outward. Later, another try at communication, excitedly,) "I'm starting medical school down at the university in two weeks!" (Jo remains unchanged. Rex, looking at her, shows concern for the first time,) "I don't mean to pry, Ma'am, but you mentioned you gave everything away and you have no things. That's a bit unusual. Your future must be assured."

Jo: (Temporarily abandoning her silence, she turns toward him, again laughs the ironic laugh,) "You surely have a way with words, Son! Yes, my future is assured." (Softly and slowly the laugh degenerates as before,) "Assured." (With a barely visible weeping, Jo resumes staring quietly out of the window.)

Rex: (Now for the first time he regards her with a frown, concerned,) "I'm sorry, Ma'am, but you seem so unhappy. Any way I can help?"

(Jo continues her mute stance, staring outwardly. He reaches over and touches her hand lightly. She withdraws in fright, staring at him, edging away.

Her tension gradually softens as time passes in silence, and she relaxes, again gazing outwardly, slowly drifting off to sleep. He continues to look at her episodically with deep concern.

They pass through a small town and stop at an intersection. Several costumed figures are soliciting for a charity-masquerade party, approaching cars at the stoplight. One figure is "Death," dressed in black with white bones painted, who jumps in front of the RV and pounds on the passenger-side windshield, holding a basket for donations. Jo awakens with a start, sees "Death" dancing in front of her, screams in horror, throws her arms around Rex, crying hysterically.)

Rex: (Calming her, his arm lightly around her,) "It's okay, just a Halloween charity trick."

Jo: (Slowly quieting down but remaining close to him, her arm around his neck,) "Death terrifies me, but I have to face it," (softly,) "face it."

Rex: "We all do at some point. But in the meantime there's a whole lot of beauty in the world. At least that's the way I see it."

Jo: (Remaining close, looking into his face, speaking in tones reflecting a complexity of tenderness, desperation and resolve; a slight smile,) "You seem a nice boy. You must have had nice parents."

Rex: (Relieved to see her gain some emotional stability, his arm still lightly about her. Laughs softly,) "Oh yes, I try to be nice." (Pause, now more seriously,) "Actually my mother died when I was born. Those things still do happen on rare occasion. My dad raised me. He's all I've ever had, and I love him dearly."

Jo: (Softly, reverently, a slight smile,) "It feels so good to be next to you. I used to hold my son closely."

Rex: "Where is he now?"

Jo: (Pause. She gradually releases him and sits staring out of the window,) "He's dead."

Rex: (Looking at her, his brow furrowed,) "What happened?" (Jo doesn't answer, resuming her immobile stance. He continues to drive along the desolate countryside, no other traffic. He glances at her frequently, frowning, concerned. They round a curve as they continue their climb.)

Jo: (Brightens slightly, points out of the window,) "Right over there, see that big plain with the mountain behind? On July 28, 1848, Captain Robert Jameson, U.S. Cavalry, led an unprovoked attack on a Sioux encampment, coming down from the mountainside at dawn. A company of thirty-six. He was angry because a Sioux half-breed girl had rebuffed him. They killed twelve Sioux with no injuries to themselves."

Rex: (Somewhat encouraged at her conversation,) "Our U.S. history has some very sad pages."

Jo: "Yes. Sadness, sadness."

Rex: "Wow, you know some stuff! What do you do?"

Jo: (Again the ironic laugh,) "Yeah, I know some stuff ." (repeating,) "Yeah." (Pause,) "I taught at the little Sioux Reservation Grade School."

Rex: "Don't teach there now?" (Jo remains silent and resumes her stationary position with outward stare.

Evening approaches, light dwindles, shadows appear, temperature dropping,) "I'm a little cool." (Zips jacket closed,) "Are you warm enough?" (Again she offers no response. Pause,) "I'm hungry. Forgot to get a snack back in town." (Glances about at the desolation and forest that surround the road they are following,) "Nothing around here and no food in the RV."

Jo: "I have a little something here." (Produces her only possession, the small paper sack,) "It's not much."

Rex: "Anything would be fine with me." (Pulls off of the road and stops the RV.)

Jo: (Opens the sack, removes a small plastic container and part of a loaf of bread,) "It's only some bread and red wine, but I'm happy to share this simple bit with you. Do you have any cups?"

Rex: "Yes, here you are." (He holds out two small plastic cups. She pours the wine from the container, reseals it and lays it aside, then breaks the bread in half, sets it between them on a napkin. She takes a cup of wine from him, holds a piece of bread, stares at the bread and wine. Silent pause, then speaking softly, barely audibly,) "This is my last -- "

Rex: "Sorry, I couldn't hear what you said."

Jo: "It's okay." (They eat and drink quietly. Jo looking at him now, and for the first time, a simple smile,) "You will become a good doctor. I can tell. Maybe you will even remember me."

Rex: "I'll remember you. I just wish I could understand you."

Jo: "Maybe you will later." (He starts the motor and pulls ahead onto the empty road, resuming their upward journey. Pause. Jo now looking out the side window attentively, speaking more strongly,) "We're almost there, a couple of miles farther. I'll show you." (Several minutes pass, the RV moving more slowly,) "There it is. See that little road off to the right? It leads into a small clearing behind the trees."

Rex: (Pulls off the road and around into a clearing and stops the RV. The scene is total desolation; heavily wooded, gathering dark clouds, temperature continues to fall,) "Ma'am, there's nothing here – perhaps a house or something deeper into the forest?"

Jo: (Laughs, a slight smile, now more settled and calm,) "Yes, there's something there." (Repeats, a more serious tone, then,) "The most beautiful scene in the world for me. All kinds of trees, birds, flowers, a rocky stream far, far below, soft breezes like caresses, a high cliff overlooking – it was religious for me, soothing. I would often go there as a child when troubled. I would pray. The natural beauty and silence and presence of God were comforting." (She moves over close to him, touches his cheek, stares deeply into his eyes. She is totally calm now, a definite smile,) "You're a good boy. I know God will bless you. You'll become a good doctor and help people in need." (Pause,) " Remember me." (Silence. She kisses him long and tenderly on the lips, climbs out of the RV, places her twenty-dollar bill on the seat,) "Take this, It's all I've got. I won't need it." (Laughs lightly but not ironically or nervously now,) "Goodbye." (She walks quickly away toward the woods.)

Rex: (Now extremely alarmed, totally realizing the mortal tragedy unfolding quickly before him, but still in control of his actions, shouts,) "No, wait, what the hell are you doing?" (In desperation, he jumps from the RV and begins to run after her, but the RV is inadequately braked and begins to roll backward. Acting reflexively, he turns and races after it, jumps in, sets the brake – now he is after her again but has lost time. Shouting desperately,) "Stop! I won't let you!"

Jo: (Now way ahead of him, laughing lightly,) "You can't stop me." (She arrives at the high cliff, stands overlooking a steep drop-off, with rocky creek far below, a deadly unbroken distance. A small but dense thicket of trees separates him from the base of her perch. The scene is one of extreme natural beauty, but by now the sky has severely darkened and rain has begun to fall; this darkness and worsening storm increases rapidly over the following sequence. Her laughter has dwindled but she remains calm. "If you come any closer, I'll jump now. I wanted to pray first, but if you come any closer I'll jump without praying."

Rex: (He stops short, now totally desperate,) "I stop! See! I stopped now! But why? Why?"

Jo: (Now crying lightly,) "Why? Because it's the only answer for me."

Rex: "Why? What answer?" (Jo's eyes are now half-closed and her lips move as she prays in inaudible tones, oblivious to his question. Rex now shouting,) "Jo, you were desperate and I helped you! I rescued you! You owe it to me to tell me -- why? What?"

Jo: (Recovering slightly, she has partially heard him, slight frown, looks toward him, speaks haltingly, unevenly,) "Desperate – helped – owe." (Then more clearly,) "Because I killed my only son. The only thing I ever loved and I killed him." (Now weeping openly.)

Rex: "No! No! I don't believe it! You couldn't kill anybody! It isn't true!"

Jo: (Speaking in even, studied tones, still crying lightly,) "As sure as if I pulled a trigger. He was into drugs. I couldn't reach him, whatever I tried or said. I was angry at him. He threatened to drive away, I pleaded for him to stay, he screamed 'No' at me. Then I said coldly, 'Okay, kid, sure! Go ahead!' I said it coldly, viciously. He stormed out the door, sped off, crashed. Because of me. I killed him. He was all I had. I loved him and I killed him. Death is the only answer for me."

Rex: (Realizing his best chance is to keep her talking,) "Wait – how old was he?"

Jo: (Sobbing,) "He was twenty-one, just a kid."

Rex: "No, he was an adult! You did all you could! He was an adult, responsible for his own actions. He made his decision, not you!" (pause,) "Why do you want to hurt me like this?"

Jo: "You?"

Rex: "Hurt me, yes, because I'm a fellow human being." (Pause, then speaking evenly and softly, frowning, a cloud of confusion momentarily crossing his face as he speaks further,) "Even more, I feel this strange attachment to you." (Pause, then more forcefully,) "And those Sioux children! They didn't do anything! Now they'll have no teacher." (Jo's eyes are half-closed now and she appears to be praying again. Pause. Rex speaks clearly, as to himself,) "Death, in front of me, on my birthday."

Jo: (Slightly recovering.) "What -- did you say?"

Rex: Jo

Rex: (Softly but matter-of-factly, his face again reflecting some confusion) "My birthday, tonight. Twenty-two years old, and here is death - again."

Jo: "Again? What – ?"

Rex: (A clouded expression again darkens his face as he speaks emotionally,) "Twenty-two years ago tonight, my mother dying as I was being born. And here's death again."

Jo: (Now confusion reflected in her face,) "Also, also, my son's birth – twenty-two years ago now." (Rex looks at her intently, takes a step toward her.) "Stop or I'll jump!"

Rex: (By now the storm has become violent, the darkness impenetrable,) "I stop! I stop!" (Pause,) "Jo! I can no longer see you!" (Strains to visualize her in the heavy downpour, wind and absolute darkness,) "Jo! Answer me! Jocasta! Please! Come back down here! For God's sake! Jo!" (Silence. Pause.

A bright lightning-flash suddenly illuminates the cliff; Rex sees that it is now empty. A flock of birds flies loudly up from far below, signifying her apparent suicide. Rex weeps bitterly as he turns and walks back to the RV, oblivious to the violent storm,) "May God have mercy on the soul of this poor misguided woman." (Pause, mumbles,) "Go back to town, get the police." (Climbs slowly into the driver's seat, turns on headlights and interior lights, looks at the twenty-dollar bill on the seat, continues bitter weeping, hair now streaked, soaking wet. Speaks slowly as a soliloquy, hands resting on the steering wheel, eyes closed, head dropped forward,) "Is this what it's going to be like to be a medical doctor? You try to help someone in trouble and you end up with death?" (Bangs his hands on the wheel,) "Damn!" (Pause, weeping, heavy rain against the windshield, thunder, wind, total darkness penetrated only by the headlights and frequent jagged lines of lightning strikes,) "But I'm going to try to become a good doctor. That's all I know to do. May God help me."

(The following is an intensely dramatic scene and must be staged carefully. Jo appears suddenly in the tumultuous storm, throws herself against the tall RV windshield directly in front of him; face turned to the side and down, eyes closed, arms outstretched with palms forward.)

Rex: "Good God!" Jumps from the cab, runs the few steps to her, arms around her waist, he lowers her slowly to the ground, cradling her in front of the headlights which emphasize the driving rain, "You're alive! You live! You came back down!" (Laughing hysterically, kissing her repeatedly on the lips, encircling her in his arms as they sit on the ground.

Jo: Opens her eyes, speaking happily yet forcefully, holding his head with both hands,) "I want you in me. I want you inside of me, where you first came into this world twenty-two years ago tonight." (Camera fades as they kiss, she still holding his head.)

(New scene, next morning, clear bright sunlight, the RV in the foreground, a doe off to the side as a sign of tranquility. Silence. After a pause showing the deer nibbling grasses, the scene shifts to inside the RV. Rex and Jo are in bed, awakening, smiling, calm.)

Jo: (On elbow, regards him,) "Awake yet?"

Rex: (Eyes half-open,) "Don't know. I'll let you know as soon as I find out."

Jo: (Pause.) "Got coffee?"

Rex: "Sure do. And I need some." (Pause.)

(Scene shifts to a small table inside the RV; both sipping coffee. Jo has a sheet draped around her, Rex in tee-shirt and shorts.)

Rex: "You okay?"

Jo: "Yes. You?"

Rex: "Okay." (They smile at each other, happy, calm. Pause,) "We have to get you back to school."

Jo: "Classes start in two weeks."

Rex: "I'll give you some money."

Jo: "I hate that."

Rex: "No – I've been working this summer. No problem. You'll need it 'til payday."

Jo: "Well, that's true, I have to get a few things." (They stare at each other. Smiles. Pause,) "You saved my life."

Rex: "No I didn't. I helped you. You saved your own life. And you affected me, in some profound way too, and now you'll be back as an important part of those Sioux Indian kids. I helped you. That's what doctors do; they help people. And, God willing, that's what I'll do the rest of my life." (Pause. She takes his hand across the table.)

Jo: "I want us always to be close."

Rex: "We will, surely."

Jo: "You said you're marrying the medical profession. That's a bit true, but still one day you'll find a girl."

Rex: (Laughs,) "I know!"

Jo: "And when that happens, you must tell me."

Rex: "You'll be the first to know. And you'll find a guy."

Jo: "Me? Old me?"

Rex: "Silly! You're not that old. And, you're smart and pretty."

Jo: "Wow! I'd better write that down!"

Rex: "Well, I guess we'd better get ready to roll. Let's see, when do I see you again? I know, my dad's coming over for Thanksgiving and I'll be out of school for a few days. Let's all plan on dining together. That's my favorite holiday! I want you to meet my father; you two will like each other, I just know." (Camera fades to transient secondary-title screen.)

Two Weeks Later

(Scene – Sioux Indian Reservation School, third grade classroom. Subtitle transiently notes this. Jo is in front of the class, with students seated at small desks.)

Jo: (Now colorfully dressed, groomed, appears happy and animated,) "So today we're going to learn something new and exciting! It's called 'sub-tract-ion.' Let's all say that word together:"

Jo and class: "Sub-tract-ion!"

Jo: "Good. Now here's what it is." (Holds up six fingers,) "How many fingers?"

Class: "Six!"

Jo: Now I'm going to sub-tract two." (Folds down two fingers,) "How many fingers left?"

Class: (Loudly,) "Four!"

Jo: "Oh, you kids! You-are-so-smart! You already know subtraction!" (Class giggles, as camera fades. Pause.)

(New scene. Camera focuses on an interior door inscribed in large letters, "Human Anatomy Laboratory. Admittance to Authorized Personnel Only." Camera shifts to inside, a large well-lit room with multiple tables, each with a human cadaver covered in semi-transparent plastic sheeting. The right arm of each cadaver is uncovered and slightly extended to the side. Four medical students sit on stools around each individual table. They wear white laboratory gowns and plastic gloves but are bare-headed. The instructor stands at a small podium and addresses the class.)

Instructor: "I'll add my welcome to you students on your first day here. As you know, we're starting with the basics: human anatomy. Initially I want to remind you that before each one of you is the physical remains of what was once a living person, just like yourselves, a person who chose to bequeath his-or-her body to you, to help you become doctors. Actually, you'd be surprised how many of these were once themselves doctors or other medical people, who chose to make this their final act toward helping fellow humans." (Pause.) "So today we take that first step of climbing a giant mountain called 'medical knowledge." (Pause,) "Pardon my poetry; something tells me I'm a better medical scientist than a poet!"

Class: (Nervous laughter.)

Instructor: "Okay, now it's time to get to work, and we'll start with the right upper extremity. Each student at the head of the table, right side, will incise from the acromio-clavicular joint anteriorly and diagonally all the way to the medial aspect of the ulnar head, exposing the biceps muscle and the neuro-vascular bundle coursing distally underneath." (Pause.) "Notice I didn't use lay terms like 'front,' 'cut', or 'side.' You're in a totally different world now, with a completely different language." (Pause,) "For many of you, this initial incision into an actual human body will be an emotional experience, and for some of you, emotionally traumatic. All I can say to you is, welcome to the world of medicine. So pick up the scalpels and go!" (Camera focuses in on Rex as he grasps his scalpel and holds it momentarily pointing upward. Camera closes in and freezes on the scalpel as credits supervene.)

The End

Screenwriter's Comments on Plot and Characters
("Trailer Talk")

A number of themes: classical, religious, psychological and philosophical interweave in this screenplay, and from multiple angles it is allegorical and rife with symbolism. Thus initially "Styx County " is a clear reference to ancient Greek mythology and the belief that the River Styx was the crossing-point of newly-dead souls into the underworld. Early on, this name predicts that a major theme of the film will be death. Obviously the film evokes Sophocles' classic Greek tragedy "Oedipus Rex," who unknowingly kills his father and marries his mother, Jocasta. In addition to the names, subtleties of association include Rex's cap with a mere hint of similarity to a crown, his golden but faded tee-shirt, and Jo's reference to him one time as "Son." As a variant of the classical Oedipus tale, here Rex kills his mother (though innocently at birth), and Jo believes she has killed her own son. But she then "marries" him (temporarily), as Rex, in her mind, has been re-identified as her son, partially by virtue of their identical birthtimes. Similarity to the Greek tale is further solidified in the last line before the epilogue, where Rex predicts the future, "I want you to meet my father. You'll like each other." In contrast to Sophocles' tragedy, here the story ends happily, in spite of the pseudo-incestuous act.

The religious association of the plot is to the last days of Christ as described in the Bible's New Testament. Thus Jo's dramatic "resurrection" as Rex's "mother", where her physical appearance on the front of the RV after her symbolic "death", evokes Christ on the cross: face turned to the side and down, eyes closed, arms outstretched with palms forward. Note her long brown hair, the headband similar to the "crown of thorns," even the darker color of her dress over the hips is suggestive of a loin-cloth. Then as Rex is holding her, their stance is reminiscent of Michelangelo's famous sculpture "Pieta", Mary holding the dead body of Christ. In addition, premonitory events to this comparison include the symbolic washing of her feet, and her "last supper."

For acting in this film, Jo's role is the most demanding. She must reveal a series of emotional states, from her initial distress at having her "final" plans thwarted, to a hysterical fear of death, to intermittent mental departures from reality, and then to a calmness as she accepts her anticipated suicide. Her "confession," which Rex has unwittingly provoked, psychologically is her life-saver: once confessed, absolution follows, guilt and remorse abate, rationality surfaces, and then serenity eventually supervenes.

Finally, after her "resurrection from death," she partially changes identity into Rex's mother, helping her relieve the burden of guilt, and subsequently she returns to psychological normality.

Rex's acting role may not be as difficult as Jo's, but nevertheless it requires depth and a level of emotional stability through intensely dramatic sequences. His growing concern and perplexity dominate the initial or travel-portion of the plot, and he later partially transforms identity into Jo's son. Her brush with death, under his care ("as a doctor,") provokes an awareness that death will at times accompany him in his future as a physician. Nevertheless he narrates an unbending conviction and resolve concerning his destiny, tempered with humility: "Doctors can help, but people save themselves."

As a philosophical statement, the film affirms existentialism. That is, one is defined as a person in life by what one does, what actions one performs, and therefore one must take responsibility for the consequences of these actions. Jo's son, not his mother, is responsible for his own death. Jo is responsible for her own decision regarding potential suicide.

Finally, after experiencing this play, the reader may wish to reflect back on its title and the role of fate in the development of its many themes.

"As you wind your way down the road of life, you may be surprised to find yourself right back at your original starting place. Then, for the very first time ever, you'll know where you are and who you are."
Ancient Oriental Proverb

? Cuban Cigars // Terminus

The preceding tale is heavy, foreboding -- even morose at times. However, I prefer to conclude this book on a lighter hue of life's many colors.

Currently most popular "literature" involving the medical scene, whether written or acted, would have us believe that hospitals are hotbeds of lust, intrigue and heavy melodrama, to wit:

"Yes, the Handsome, Brilliant, Young Plastic Surgeon, only two years out of Medical School and already the Darling of Hollywood Celebrities and International Royalty, faced his greatest challenge! The scalpel was light and unswerving in his powerful grip as he worked feverishly – (even though he'd been operating for eighteen hours straight!) This incredibly difficult case had been rejected by all others: repairing the badly mangled fingers of the Famous Classical Pianist (who had been run over by a freight train). Would this Handsome, Brilliant Young Musician be able to make his scheduled, sold-out Hollywood Bowl Debut only two weeks hence, to introduce his newest composition titled: *Air, Water and Dirt*; A Triple-Concerto in C-Flat Minor for Solo Piano?

The Handsome, Brilliant Young Surgeon was CONFIDENT!

And all the while the Beautiful Blond Assistant Resident, standing close beside him and firmly holding his Instrument, could hardly contain herself as she gazed, Longingly, Aadoringly, Lustfully, into his piercing grey-green Eyes, just visible over his blood-spattered Surgical Mask, his Forehead beaded with Perspiration beneath the searing operating room Lights.

– It was three AM."

Nein! Negativo! Not.

But real drama does appear sporadically about the actual hospital scene, jumping out often unexpectedly and unannounced among the daily chores – a few would use the term "drudgery" – of routine medical work. In these pages I have attempted to portray, in both fiction and non-, some of these more compelling themes. Okay, I admit straying transiently at times onto other (barely) related realms. I hope for success in piquing the reader's interest into this truly dramatic, but mostly hidden, medical arena.

Still, some lighter-side fanciful "stuff" does happen occasionally there on the hospital wards, and one such true tale is suitable for the conclusion of this volume.

189

Toward the end of 1982, I was tidying-up my paper-work at University Hospital, preparing for a year's leave-of-absence in Saudi Arabia, to help with their evolving medical care and educational systems. Writing notes in patients' charts at the workstation of our Myocardial Infarction Research Unit ("MIRU," scene of monumental research in acute heart attack treatment), I had paid scant attention to an announcement that we had recently hired some additional foreign employees. But then I noticed a new attractive dark-haired nurse, animated. My first reaction was, "She looks Cuban." Then a second thought followed quickly, "Wow, maybe a source of Cuban rum, or even Cuban cigars!"

We had several dates before my leaving for the Middle East. (It turned out she wasn't Cuban after all, but rather Cajun, from south Louisiana. "Oh well, I got the first letter right, anyway." So I was deprived of rum and cigars, but instead she proved a source of some of the best food in the world.)

Departing, I phoned her from the airport.
"Oh, I didn't think you'd call."

She wrote to me every day for a year.

I recalled Homer's ancient Greek epic, The Odyssey, wherein the hero's wife, Penelope, waits twenty years for his return from the Trojan War. Now one isn't exactly twenty, but the principle is the same. Furthermore I didn't slay dozens of her suitors upon return home, as did the great warrior-King, Odysseus, assisted by his son, using arrows, spears, axes and bare hands. But had there been any around, I would have been tempted.

We courted another seventeen years before wedding. ("Hey!" My dear departed mother had warned long ago, "Don't rush into things!" "Okay!") Even in marrying, there were a few odd twists of fate: to avoid family inconveniences, we eloped, the only other aware of our secret plan was a close friend, a Catholic Monsignor. I again recalled the classics, *Romeo and Juliet,* wherein the only accomplice in their complex plot to join and survive was the village priest. But unlike the play's tragic end (the final line: "Never was writ a sadder tale of woe, than that of Juliet and her Romeo.") our post-nuptial path has proceeded happily.

So rather than a reception, we had a standard (?!) New Orleans party (a disguised announcement event) with a courtyard full of best friends, none of whom had the slightest notion we'd ever marry after all those years. I had a short, funny follow-up speech prepared, but never had a chance to deliver it – the simple announcement was as a bomb exploding! Every female burst into tears; every male screamed! Total chaos!

Only later was I permitted to convey my comic explanation of our matrimony: "Through these seventeen years I'd often ask, 'Shouldn't we marry?' And she'd always answer, 'But we're so young, so innocent!' And I'd concur, 'Well, that's true.' Then as the years passed and I got my hearing aid, developed cataracts, went on Medicare and retired, we agreed we weren't exactly young anymore. (Now the question of innocence is still being debated!)"

As a final-final word, I invite readers to contact me regarding this book, negative or pos'. I do believe most would agree, "It's different." Write me at www.baxbook.com. I'll read each and post the good ones, con or pro.

Cheers and all the best to you! – Bax

"Out through the fields and the woods,
    And over the walls I have wended,
I have climbed the hills of view,
    And looked at the world, and descended;
I have come by the highway home,
    And lo, it is ended."

Robert Frost
(American Poet, 1874-1963)

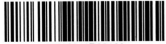

Made in the USA
Lexington, KY
04 October 2018